EQUINOX
THE BRAIN

EQUINOX
THE BRAIN

JACK CHALLONER

First published in 2000 by Channel 4 Books, an imprint of Macmillan
Publishers Ltd, 25 Eccleston Place, London SW1W 9NF and Basingstoke.

www.macmillan.co.uk

Associated companies throughout the world.

ISBN 0 7522 2326 7

Text © Jack Challoner, 2000

The right of Jack Challoner to be identified as the author of this work has
been asserted by him in accordance with the Copyright, Designs and
Patents Act 1988.

9 7 5 3 1 2 4 6 8

A CIP catalogue record for this book is available from the British Library.

Design by Jane Coney
Typeset by Ferdinand Pageworks
Printed in Great Britain by Mackays of Chatham plc

ACKNOWLEDGEMENTS

Many people have helped me to write this book. Friends and family – in particular Paula James, Carolyn McGoldrick, Daniel Brookman, Karen Darling and Jilly Duckworth – have been supportive as ever. I would like to thank Emma Tait at Channel 4 Books, and my editor Christine King, for their professionalism and enthusiasm. I would also like to acknowledge the makers of the *Equinox* series for communicating issues of contemporary science and contributing to the public understanding of the subject.

PRODUCTION CREDITS

Mind Readers
accompanies the *Equinox* programme of the same name made
by Illuminations Television Limited for Channel 4.
First broadcast: 1 December 1997

Natural-born Genius
accompanies the *Equinox* programme of the same name made
by John Gau Productions for Channel 4.
First broadcast: 3 November 1997

Phantom Brains
accompanies the *Equinox* programme of the same name made
by Oxford Television Limited for Channel 4.
First broadcast: 7 June 1999

Living Dangerously
accompanies the *Equinox* programme of the same name made
by TVF for Channel 4.
First broadcast: 12 April 1999

Thin Air
accompanies the *Equinox* programme of the same name made
by WGBH/*NOVA*
Research cited in this chapter is drawn from 'Alive on Everest',
a *NOVA* Online Adventure.
www.pbs.org/wgbh/nova/everest/expeditions/97/index.html
First broadcast: 11 August 1998

Lies and Delusions
accompanies the programme of the same name made by
Rosetta Pictures for Channel 4.
First broadcast: 28 February 2000 and 6 March 2000

CONTENTS

INTRODUCTION

Everything you experience, you experience because of your brain. All your thoughts and dreams; your perception of yourself and the world around you; that indescribable sense of awareness; your memories – all these are created by the wet, interconnected grey and white lumps inside your skull.

The scientific study of the brain provides us with insight into the very nature of ourselves, and attempts to solve one of the most important puzzles of science and philosophy: just how does the brain work? This scientific endeavour has many different branches – some of the main areas are investigated in this book. Each chapter, based on subjects covered by Channel 4's *Equinox* series, provides different pieces of the puzzle, producing a clearer picture of the brain. I have been able to extend the scope of the television programmes, and to present the science, history, philosophy and politics of these very human stories in greater detail.

Of the various branches of neuroscience (the all-encompassing term for the scientific study of the brain), neurophysiology is the attempt to work out how the structures of the brain and nervous system actually function: how they communicate with each other to endow us with the powers of thought, language, memory and perception. Neurology is very similar, but focuses more on the diagnosis and treatment of brain damage or disorder, such as epilepsy and the effects of strokes. Both neurology and neurophysiology have been organized, sophisticated areas of study for more than a hundred years. Relative newcomers to the field are neuro-chemistry – the study of the brain's chemical environment – and behavioural genetics, which aims to discover whether any aspects of our behaviour are inherited. Psychology – the study of mind and behaviour – is also part of the study of the brain, by virtue of the fact that as far as we know the mind is produced by the brain. Psychology has made great strides in fathoming human behaviour, but there is still a gulf between an understanding of the brain that produces the mind and the behaviour that the mind produces.

The human brain is incredibly complicated – the most complex object known. However, its basic structure can be described fairly easily. It has distinct areas, each of which is connected to many others. The most obvious feature is the cerebrum, the familiar convoluted grey structure that obscures the rest of the brain. It consists of two cerebral hemispheres – although the brain is not quite spherical – which are connected by a thick bridge of nerve fibres deep inside. The wrinkled surface layer of the cerebrum is the cortex, consisting of thousands of millions of interconnect-ed neurones. The neurone is the fundamental unit of the brain. Neurones produce or conduct electrical impulses that are the basis of sensation, memory, thought and motor signals that make muscles work to produce move-ment. There are other types of cell present, but they only give support and nourishment to these cellular workhorses. Neurones are like other cells in many ways: they have a nucleus and a membrane, for example. However, they dif-fer in the way they function. A neurone has long fibres, called axons, coming from its cell body. Emanating from an axon or from the cell body itself are other, smaller fibres called dendrites. Neurones communicate with each other: electrical signals pass along the axon and the dendrites, and the brain is constantly buzzing with these signals. The matter that makes up the cortex is grey, distinct from the white matter that makes up the bulk of the cerebral hemispheres it surrounds.

Beneath the all-encompassing cerebrum are other, smaller, parts of the brain, also composed of neurones. In the middle of the brain there is a cluster of smaller structures: the basal ganglia, the thalamus and hypothalamus, and the limbic system. Unlike the cerebrum, we share these structures with all other vertebrates, and this suggests they are involved in some kind of automatic processing. In fact these structures seem to be involved in the production of emotional responses, necessary for automatic reactions to fear, for example. Tucked underneath the back of the cerebrum is a cauliflower-shaped 'little brain' – the cerebellum. This sits at the top of the brainstem, which connects the brain to the top of the spinal cord.

The brain has not always been held as the centre of human thought. Most of the ancient Greek anatomists and natural philosophers, for example, believed that thinking and feeling took place in the heart or the lungs. They saw the brain more as the 'seat of the soul'. However, as early as the sixth century BC the Greek philosopher Pythagoras suggested that the brain was the organ of the mind. The Greek physician Herophilus of Chalcedon realized that the brain is the centre of the nervous system, and several other Greek thinkers began to recognize the importance of the brain in perception, thought and movement. But the brain was to remain a total mystery for many hundreds of years. During the second century AD the influential Graeco-Roman anatomist Galen of Pergamum made many important advances in the study of the nervous system. He carried out ground-breaking experiments – mainly on animals – in an attempt to understand how the human body works. For example, in one of many experiments on live animals he demonstrated that the brain controls the voice, by tying off one of the nerves that connects the brain to the larynx. Galen also correctly surmised the existence of sensory and motor nerve fibres. Despite his many useful contributions to medical science, and to anatomy and physiology in particular, many of Galen's theories were misguided or simply wrong, but they survived more or less unchallenged for 1,500 years.

During the late Middle Ages, the ideas of the ancient Greeks were modified or extended. Many people believed, for example, that the three main ventricles of the brain (those spaces filled with cerebrospinal fluid) were each responsible for a different aspect of brain function: sensation, reason and memory. During the sixteenth and seventeenth centuries, the long-standing ideas of Galen and his contemporaries, as well as the misguided modifications of the Middle Ages, were challenged by the eager endeavours of Renaissance scientists. Anatomists and physiologists, mainly in Italy, began a complete overhaul of the understanding of the brain. One by one, the various parts of the brain were identified – although, of course, knowledge of their functions was very limited. The nature of the grey and white matter was also uncovered: in the 1660s the Italian anatomist Marcello Malpighi became the first person ever to see, under a microscope, the neurones that make up the cerebrum. And at the end of the eighteenth century another Italian anatomist, Luigi Galvani, demonstrated that nerve impulses are electrical. In a series of classic experiments, he made the muscles of frogs' legs twitch by stimulating them with static electricity. His observations led him to postulate the existence of 'animal electricity'. This was the beginning of the modern understanding of how neurones work – but only in the past eighty years or so have neuroscientists been able to understand the details of how nerve impulses are generated.

Today, science is well on the way to explaining how the brain functions. To date, it has worked out how the different structures and regions within the brain are interconnected. It has shown which parts of the brain are important in various tasks, such as remembering, feeling sad, reading, using grammar or looking at something. And it has uncovered the biological and biochemical processes that underlie all the electrical signals that make up our thoughts, movements, memories and emotions. Despite these impressive advances, though, neuroscience is still in its infancy. For example, we do not yet understand in detail how the electrical signals in the nervous system actually create thoughts, memories and emotions. The pathways of perception and the production of movement are fairly well understood and in great detail, but little is known about how movement and perception actually relate to our conscious awareness. Just how our brains make us aware at all is a mystery that is not likely to be worked out for some time, if ever. Consciousness may turn out to be one of those fundamental, elusive phenomena – like the ultimate origin of space and time – that science may never fully explain.

This does not mean that the journey towards understanding it is a waste of time. At each step along the way, new wonders and mysteries become apparent. Besides, the study of the brain is not restricted to finding answers to ultimate questions. It is carried out as much with medical goals in mind as with scientific or philosophical ones, and each advance in neurophysiology brings new hope to those suffering from disorders of the brain, whether caused by physical damage or disease.

Of the various branches of neuroscience, neurophysiology, neurology and behavioural genetics are all in the spotlight in 'Mind Readers', which looks at the origin of social aspects of behaviour, such as the ability to empathize. Neurophysiologists have begun to work out which parts of the brain contribute to our social awareness, but neurologists are involved, too: social behaviours can be impaired in certain mental disorders, including autism. People with autism find it difficult to relate to other people, and to understand why people behave as they do. The chapter ends by considering the genetic factors involved in our social behaviour. 'Natural-born Genius' considers the nature of human intelligence, and involves psychology and behavioural genetics. The study of the nature of intelligence, and attempts to measure it, are tasks of the psychologists, but it has long been wondered whether a person's intelligence is determined by his or her genetic makeup. As will become clear, philosophy and politics are never far from the debate about intelligence. 'Phantom Brains' explores a neurological phenomenon that was once no more than a medical curiosity – but that now helps to give new insights into how the brain produces a body image, a sense of self. That phenomenon is the vivid sensation felt by an amputee that the lost limb is still present. New theories to explain this 'phantom' sensation are challenging some long-held beliefs about the brain. The subject of 'Living Dangerously' is the origin of thrill-seeking behaviour. What makes people want to take risks, and why do some take more risks than others? Many people today believe that mind and behaviour are produced by electrical signals and chemical reactions in their brain, and it turns out that the chemical environment of the brain may be related to a person's desire for risk. This situation suggests a kind of biochemical fate – as if we have no control over our behaviour. This is a recurrent theme in neuroscience: an example of the nature versus nurture debate.

Another recurrent theme of neuroscience is the use of new developments in technology, which help to achieve breakthroughs at an ever increasing speed. For example, new brain-imaging techniques are helping neurologists in their diagnoses and helping neurophysiologists to test their theories about how the brain works. These imaging techniques include MRI (magnetic resonance imaging) and PET (positron emission tomography). They are non-invasive – there is no need to open up a person's head to study the living brain – and produce clear visual representations of brain activity. Scanning techniques rely heavily on computing power, and computers are important in neuroscience in other ways. All scientists have benefited from the information age: they can collect and analyse data more quickly and efficiently, and can communicate their results effectively using computers. But computers are useful to neuroscience in other ways. They are being used to model the way individual brain cells – neurones – work together to achieve memory and learning. Truly intelligent computer systems, which can think for themselves, may be the ultimate result of such research but, for now, computer models of how the brain works are helping to test the latest theories.

The brain is so vital to us that we can easily take its amazing capabilities for granted. 'Thin Air' demonstrates what happens to the brain when it begins to run low on energy, as we follow a scientific expedition to the summit of Mount Everest. 'Lies and Delusions' looks at some of the most bizarre symptoms investigated by neurologists, including claims made by patients whose brains have been damaged in such a way that they think their parents are impostors. It is specific damage to the outer surface of the brain – the cortex that surrounds the walnut-shaped cerebral hemisphere of the brain – that causes these strange symptoms. Study of the effects of damage to the cortex is helping to reveal the way the brain works. Finally, a brief Afterword looks ahead to the fascinating future of developments in neuroscience.

MIND READERS
...in search of the social brain...

Most human beings are mind readers: we can often tell what people are feeling without asking them. You could call this amazing ability a sixth sense, but as far as we know this is no mystical quality – not a kind of telepathy, for example. Instead, mind reading seems to be a facet of the normal functioning of the human brain: we can see beyond people's eyes, and engage with the minds that lie behind them. Neuroscientists believe that various parts of the brain work together to enable us to sense what other people are feeling – to empathize with them. These brain components, working together in this way, are sometimes referred to as the 'social brain'. The varied tools of modern neuroscience are helping scientists to find out what those components are, and to begin to understand how the social brain works.

Can you mind read?
To give you an example of the mind-reading capabilities of the social brain, imagine watching the following scene. A man standing at a bus stop is approached from behind by a woman who thinks she recognizes him. The woman taps the man on the shoulder but, as he turns around, she realizes that she does not know him after all, and rushes away looking embarrassed. Most people watching this scene would easily work out what is going on, by observing the woman's and the man's reactions. We are able to 'get

inside' the minds of the two people involved. As far as we know, this ability to empathize sets humans apart from all other animals.

An important part of this skill is the way we interpret facial expressions. When shown a photograph of an expressive face, most people can recognize the emotion being expressed at the moment the photograph was taken. Even if the photograph shows only a person's eyes, it is normally possible to identify what they are feeling: eyes can reveal joy, anxiety, sadness or disinterest, for example. Simon Baron-Cohen, at the University of Cambridge, is determined to find out how the social brain works, and how it relates to disorders such as autism as well as to differences between men and women. He and his team have put together a set of pictures of facial expressions for use in his tests and, as he says, 'Sometimes when an emotional expression changes ... the whole face changes. But often, changes in emotion are much more subtle, and you may not see a big change in the mouth, but you may see a very subtle change in what goes on around the eyes. We appear, as mind readers, to be very skilled in picking up these minute changes.'

Some people refer to eyes as the 'windows to the soul'; reading another person's eyes plays a major role in our ability to empathize. Other primates – chimpanzees, for example – seem to communicate using facial expressions. However, it is unlikely that the interpretation of faces is as sophisticated in chimpanzees as in humans. And unlike all other social animals – from ants to elephants and including chimpanzees – we engage each other in meaningful conversation and, perhaps more crucially, understand that others have their own views on the world and their own feelings. This helps us to act in a manner appropriate to a particular situation.

When you think about it, social interaction is sensitive and extremely complex. Our brains are constantly bombarded by sensory information – from our eyes, ears and nose, from touch and taste, from pain receptors – and are somehow able to act on this information. What actually goes on in the brain during a social interaction – for example, when we meet someone for the first time? First, the brain must evaluate what is going on. To do this, we analyse the behaviour of others: their facial expressions, their body language, their tone of voice. This kind of response involves our emotions, which are, at least in part, automatic functions of the brain. It has been shown that our body responds to emotional stimuli even when we are unaware of what the stimuli are: the heart rate quickens or we sweat in fearful situations, for example. This kind of reflex action is particularly important in frightening or novel situations. Once the brain has generated this kind of response, it elicits an action: it must interpret, or experience, the emotion. Based on this experience, the brain must then produce an output in the form of appropriate behaviour. This third stage involves our intelligence and our memories. The appropriate behaviour in a particular situation may be to hold back – it is not always acceptable to say the first thing that comes into our heads, for example. People who are unable to hold back are perceived as impulsive and insensitive – antisocial – rather than tactful and intuitive, with an active social brain.

So the social brain probably consists of a few distinct functions – perhaps even three distinct structures within the brain. If we are to unravel the mysteries of the social brain, we must first locate parts of the brain that are involved in our emotions, then parts of the brain that make us aware of what is going on, and then parts that generate the appropriate action.

One clue to the whereabouts of the elements of the social brain might be the fact that some people are better at mind reading than others – they have more effective social brains. By comparing the brains of different people and relating them to psychological observation and evaluation, significant differences might show up. These differences might reveal the source of our social behaviour.

Sexual stereotypes?

What kinds of people are more sociable than others? There seems to be a perception that women are generally more intuitive and sensitive than men, for example. This would involve a very active social brain: a vivid ability to mind read. How does this relate to stereotypes, such as the idea that women spend their time discussing each other's feelings, and take caring jobs such as nursing or teaching? The fact that there actually are more women than men in caring professions must be at least partly due to the very existence of these stereotypes: the result of social expectations and history. But is there an element of truth behind the stereotypes? Are women really better mind readers? Psychological tests indicate that, generally, they are. When, for example, women are shown photographs of faces, they are generally better than men at identifying the emotion being expressed. Of course, these tests might simply be illustrating the very stereotypes they attempt to look beyond. For by analysing the behaviour of adult women, researchers are recording the behaviour of brains that have been developing over many years, all the time surrounded by a world in which there is pressure to 'fit in'. You could ask: 'Do women tend to be more intuitive just because that's what women do?' The obvious approach to overcome this test bias is to study the behaviour of very young babies, who are as yet unaffected by society's role modelling. There does seem to be a large body of evidence that apparently supports the idea that females naturally have different approaches to social situations from men.

There have been many books in recent years that have analysed the differences between men and women. This is partly a reaction to the way in which gender roles have shifted so dramatically over the past hundred years or so, and partly a result of interesting new discoveries and ideas in physiology, biochemistry and psychology. In *Brain Sex: The Real Difference Between Men and Women*, authors Anne Moir and David Jessel lay bare what seem like innate differences between men and women. They report some amazing and consistent findings. For example, girls are considerably more sensitive to touch and to sound at just a few hours old. Girl babies generally respond better to emotional speech, and are more easily calmed down by a soothing voice. At a very early age, girl babies are more interested in communicating with other people than boys, who tend to be more interested in inanimate objects. These differences in behaviour between babies of the opposite sex may be the purest signs of differences in the social brain, before social conditioning can have any effect. But there is evidence that the differences in the social brains of girls and boys do underlie the behaviour of adults, too. Another book about differences between the sexes, *Sex on the Brain: The Biological Differences Between Men and Women* by Deborah Blum, tells us an amazing tale of gender confusion in Dominica in the West Indies. Some families there pass on a gene that makes young boys appear to be female – even down to the genitals – until they are in their early teens, at the onset of puberty. Then, what looks like a large clitoris swiftly becomes a penis and, where once there was nothing, two normal, healthy, sperm-producing testicles drop down. These children are raised as girls because, until the changes appear, they look like girls. As soon as it is realized that they are male, the boys apparently begin to make the switch to 'typical male behaviour' without too much fuss.

So it seems that there is a biological basis to differences between male and female behaviours: the two sexes do seem to be fundamentally different from each other. Perhaps women really are generally more sensitive than men. Does that mean that men are unsociable, unable to mind read? There are certainly countless stories of men being insensitive or uncaring; unable to read people's minds. Again, this is certainly not true of every man, but most people would more readily associate lack of sensitivity with men than with women. And the male brain's perceived greater interest in physical objects than in people also seems to persist into adulthood – again, in general. Meet Chris: he is what some people might call a typical 'nerd'. He works with computers, and has always had an interest in electronics and all things technical. As a boy, he spent far more time with his chemistry set than with people. More recently, he has reorganized the family's compact disc collection according to the dates of birth of the composers, and he regularly joins in competitions in which the sole aim is to contact as many people as possible on his citizen band radio over a twenty-four-hour period. More importantly, Chris has never really had many friends, and finds it hard to function in social situations. His wife Gisele says that he is not at all good at gauging when she is upset. Often, when he comes through the door after a day at work, he will not think to say hello to her, perhaps assuming that having heard the door slam she will know he has returned.

'These things – you just tend to accept them and think they are eccentricities,' says Gisele. 'And yet, thinking back, it's quite strange to lie down and go to sleep at social occasions ... I have learned that I have to tell him when I'm upset, and precisely why.'

If women really are better at reading social cues, how might we explain the difference? Human behaviour is extremely complex, and is no doubt shaped by a huge number of factors, many of them probably far too subtle ever to be fully understood. But where behaviour differs in a general sense between the sexes, can science identify the underlying causes of that difference? If women are born mind readers and men are born nerds, then we should find some physiological differences between men and women – but where might we find this evidence? Our mind-reading capability comes from our brain, so perhaps a man's brain is different from a woman's. Physiological difference between males and females is called sex dimorphism: is there any sex dimorphism in the brain that might account for the different social behaviours of men and women?

Sex and sensitivity

As we grow, the connections between neurones in our brains strengthen or weaken, and new ones are created, as we lay down memories and learn from our experiences. So the brains of any two people differ, because everyone has different experiences. This difference at neurone level does affect our behaviour, and could account for some of the differences between the 'typical' behaviours of men and women. This will be particularly true where male and female roles are well defined, and developing children are expected to follow them. In this case, women who have broadly similar experiences could develop similar nerve pathways in the brain. But these neural pathways are too small to be detected, and will differ from person to person and between different cultures. Are there any sex dimorphisms that occur consistently enough to explain the perceived ability of women to have a more finely tuned social brain than men? Neuroscientists do not have enough evidence to give a definite answer to this, although during the past twenty years or so more and more sex dimorphisms have been reported. One of the best-known examples concerns the corpus callosum, a bundle of nerve fibres that connects the two hemispheres of the brain. In 1982 cell biologist Christine De Lacoste-Utamsing and anthropologist Ralph Holloway found that certain regions of the corpus callosum were significantly larger in women than in men. Their result has been disputed in several more recent studies. In some experiments, involving rats, it has even been found that the corpus callosum grows larger under the influence of male hormones.

The corpus callosum, like most other structures of the brain, is composed of neurones that carry electrical signals. But the brain is alive with chemical as well as electrical messages. Among them are hormones. An orchestra of hormones, largely produced in or directed by the brain, is carried by the blood, and can have effect quickly, efficiently and body-wide. Many hormones are released by the pituitary gland, including those that affect growth, the conservation of water by the body and the amount of sugar our cells 'burn' to obtain energy. Hormones help to regulate our bodies, but they can also affect our minds. They can influence our mood, inducing anxiety or producing pleasurable feelings. Might hormones have a role in the social brain?

Sex hormones account for the physical differences between men and women. The main group of female sex hormones, oestrogens, help to cause the growth of breasts during puberty, as well as more structural differences such as a wider pelvis and shorter vocal cords. Similarly, the main male sex hormone, testosterone, causes development of the male sex organs, and causes men to grow more body hair than women. But can they account for sex dimorphism in the social brain, and for the differing behaviour of men and women? Some studies, mainly in animals, have shown that oestrogens make a female more sexually active during her most fertile times, while testosterone has long been known to affect behaviour – increasing 'macho' actions, violent tendencies and sex drive in men.

In 1959 neuroscientist Charles Barraclough found startling evidence of the roles of sex hormones, while carrying out experiments on rats at the University of California, Los Angeles. He injected female rats with testosterone while they were still in their mothers' wombs, and found that the rats grew up permanently sterile, unable to ovulate. More interestingly, they adopted behaviours typical of male rats. In fact, female rats injected with testosterone were found to mount other, unaltered females. This kind of observation led to theories about another facet of behaviour: sexual orientation. Some studies in the 1970s found levels of testosterone in gay men were lower than in heterosexual men. These studies are now largely discredited – one of them included bisexual men, who were found to have higher levels of testosterone than either heterosexual or gay men. Nevertheless, hormones might have an important role in the social brain.

Also during the 1970s, several studies showed sex dimorphism in certain structures in the brains of rats. In particular, parts of the hypothalamus were larger or more densely populated with neurones in females than in males, while other parts were smaller or less dense. One of these sites was actually named the sexually dimorphic nucleus. The hypothalamus is the controller of many hormones, including those released by the pituitary gland. Among these pituitary hormones are those that trigger the release of sex hormones from the testes or the ovaries. The hypothalamus, right at the centre of the head, has long been associated with many different human behaviours. It has a mass of only about ten grams (a third of an ounce), but it has been shown to have major roles in regulating body temperature, controlling thirst and appetite, and influencing blood pressure, sexual behaviour, aggression, fear and sleep. And sex dimorphism in the hypothalamus has been found in human brains, just as in rats' brains.

It seems that there are several differences between men's and women's brains. Might differences in sex hormones, the hypothalamus or the corpus callosum account for women's supposed superior mind-reading capabilities? Although our hormones do affect our behaviour, it is unlikely that their differing levels can be responsible for the sex dimorphism of the social brain. The secretion of hormones by the body changes with temperature, over time and with age – it is not constant enough to explain why women are consistently better at mind reading. Studies of the corpus callosum have not shown consistent differences between men and women. And as yet, reading social cues is one of the few tasks with which the hypothalamus has not been linked: it is associated with control over body maintenance, rather than the subtleties of mind reading.

Comparing the anatomy of the brains of men and women is daunting, and has so far proved inconclusive when it comes to the social brain. Is there another way that we might be able to unravel its workings? Can we pin down which parts of the brain are involved in basic mind-reading tasks, such as interpreting a facial expression? Modern brain-scanning techniques, along with some scientific detective work, have begun to do just this, and neuroscientists are beginning to understand how the social brain works. As we shall see, the amygdalae and the orbitofrontal cortex have been identified as two of the main parts of the social brain. This is a fascinating quest in itself, but it may also benefit the study of autism. People with autism live in a frustrating, closed world. Their social skills are generally impaired, and they seem unable or unwilling to take other people's feelings into account. Indeed, Chris the 'nerd' has recently been diagnosed as having a mild form of autism, called Asperger's syndrome. This diagnosis, along with the better understanding of how the autistic brain works, has helped Chris and his wife Gisele come to terms with his lack of social awareness that has plagued their relationship and even threatened to destroy it. Are there any links between autism and typical male behaviour, including the behaviour of the social brain? Might we be able to obtain clues as to the functioning of the normal social brain by studying the brains of people with autism? The answer might just be yes.

All alone
The word 'autism' – meaning 'aloneness' – was first used in 1912 by Swiss psychologist Eugen Bleuler to refer to the

inner world of schizophrenics. It was chosen as the name for the disorder that we know as autism by the scientist who first identified the condition in 1943 – American Leo Kanner at the Johns Hopkins Children's Psychiatric Clinic in Baltimore, USA. Kanner identified a set of characteristics that he had observed in a group of his patients, including the characteristic aloneness and a desire for routine. A year later – but independently of Kanner – a Swiss physician, Hans Asperger, described the same set of symptoms, and also used the word 'autism'. Both these scientists believed that the medical condition they had described was present from birth. Their contemporaries considered the symptoms of autism to be the result of bad parenting, since the disorder does not become evident until the child is three or four years old. As we shall see, this is when the development of the social brain in children is becoming apparent.

Most neuroscientists estimate that some form of autism is found in one in every five or six hundred people. This means that in the UK more than a hundred thousand people have autism; in the USA almost six hundred thousand. It is difficult to obtain an accurate estimate, because not everyone has exactly the same set of symptoms. In fact the medical community now considers autism to be one of a range of related conditions, known collectively as PDDs (pervasive developmental disorders). These are 'spectrum disorders', meaning that their symptoms can be anything from moderate to severe. The most severe cases can be somewhat distressing: such people are frustratingly locked away inside their own minds; their language is seriously impaired; they have much lower than average general intelligence; and they often make repetitive physical motions such as rocking to and fro. People whose symptoms lie towards the moderate end of the spectrum are often diagnosed as having Asperger's syndrome. People with this syndrome, like those with more severe autistic symptoms, are less able than most people to empathize and to be sociable. But in contrast, their language is normally more or less unaffected, and their intelligence as measured by standard IQ (intelligence quotient) is often above average. Such people can lead a normal life, to the extent that they may not be diagnosed as having the syndrome until they are adults – that is what happened to Chris.

In the past ten years, a good deal of research has been carried out into the causes of autism. As well as the behavioural aspects of the disorder, it has been found that people with autism often have other symptoms in common. These include a dietary problem called 'leaky gut' and elevated levels of a neurotransmitter called serotonin. In leaky gut, protein molecules that would normally pass straight through the digestive system are absorbed into the blood through the intestinal wall. Some of these proteins, such as casein, found in milk, can break down in the blood to form substances that act like opium. Certain behavioural aspects of autism – including perhaps the characteristic 'aloneness' – might be connected with the effects of these substances on the brain. The same aspects might also be attributed to the higher than normal levels of serotonin. People with schizophrenia, a disorder that shares some features with autism, have a similar imbalance of serotonin. Leaky gut and imbalances of neurotransmitter might be to blame for some of the effects of autism, though what causes them is another question. Because the disorder is a syndrome – meaning that sufferers have some or all of a collection of symptoms – it probably has a number of different causes. A small proportion of the cases of autism can be shown to be caused by rubella (German measles) during pregnancy. Genetics may ultimately be the cause of most cases, however. Families in which one member has autism are more likely to see occurrence in subsequent children than other families. Siblings are significantly more likely both to have autism if they are twins than if they are not. As autism has many symptoms, you would expect that it is caused by abnormalities in several genes. In 1997, the first of these genes was identified. Researchers at the University of Chicago investigated eighty-six children with autism and found that all of them had an abnormal version of a gene that is responsible for the transportation of serotonin around the body.

So much for the possible causes of autism. What are people with autism like? How do they experience the world? Perhaps the most famous person with autism was a fictional one: Raymond Babbitt, played by Dustin Hoffman in the 1989 film *Rain Man*. In Hoffman's sensitive, Oscar-winning portrayal of Raymond, he illustrates some of the characteristics that are common to many people with autism. Raymond is not interested in other people, or in how they are feeling. Like many autistic people, he has exceptional arithmetical skills. Although people with autism often have lower than average general intelligence, it is not uncommon for them to have amazing skills of computation – mental arithmetic – or incredible memories for facts and figures. Many autistic people are able to carry out different but equally remarkable computational tasks: playing a piece of music note for note after hearing it just once, or producing accurate drawings of a scene they saw just once, for example. In *Rain Man*, Raymond's hustling brother Charlie cynically takes advantage of his arithmetical ability; but Raymond is unaware of being used. This, too, is a common characteristic of people with autism: because they are unable to understand that other people can feel differently about things – they are unable to empathize – they easily fall prey to the most straightforward pranks or confidence tricks.

People with autism live in a closed world. Alison Gopnik, at the University of California, Berkeley, gives an insight into their perceptions: 'What they're seeing is a bag of skin ... stuffed into clothes, draped over pieces of furniture, with these two little dots on top that are moving back and forth, and this hole underneath that opens and closes and has noises coming out. You can imagine how terrifying, how unpredictable, how confusing it would be to make sense of what these bags of skin are doing.' Confusion and anxiety lead to antisocial or solitary behaviour. While most other schoolchildren are busy playing games with each other, sharing experiences, children with autism are spending most of their time with their own thoughts, investigating not the people but the objects around them.

Children with autism mostly attend special schools, where teachers can provide them with the most appropriately stimulating, and understanding, environment. The most able children can be taught what to look out for in order to interpret what other people might be feeling, to help them survive in a confusing world. Alec, Josh and Robert are such children. They sit around a classroom table, looking at photographs in which other children are expressing obvious emotions. But the boys are bewildered by what they see. They are shown a photograph of a girl who is clearly looking very upset because she has fallen off her bicycle. When asked what the boys think the girl in the picture is feeling, they try to analyse what has happened, and to work out logically, rather than emotionally, how that might make the girl feel. So Josh says – after a long pause – 'I think the girl is unhappy, because she has fallen off her bike.' Josh was not able to get an immediate sense of the sadness of the girl by looking at the expression on her face.

Learning about human behaviour in this way – as if it was in a textbook – is like observing an alien species. The title of Oliver Sacks' book, *An Anthropologist on Mars*, aptly sums up how adults with autism often describe growing up. The title chapter of that book describes the life of Temple Grandin, a professor of animal science at Colorado State University. Grandin does not feel love or compassion: she finds it almost impossible to empathize. Like many people with autism, her overriding emotion is fear. A large proportion of the abattoirs in the USA are built according to designs worked out by Grandin. She can understand the behaviour of cows better than she can understand human behaviour. She interacts quite naturally with them – explaining that fear is their main emotion, too. Her ranch and abattoir designs are therefore among the most humane. Grandin compares herself to Mr Spock in *Star Trek*, and refers to non-autistic people as 'emotibots', who function according to feelings rather than reason alone. As she grew up she realized that, unlike her own, other people's thoughts and actions were related to their feelings. Unlike people who do not have autism – who have insight into social behaviour and are able to engage with other people's minds – Grandin has had to work out how other people form and retain relationships, by observing but not participating. She calls other people's normal social interactions ISPs (interesting sociological phenomena). She describes her mind as a network of supercomputers, filled with experiences and observations stored over many years. In any situation, she downloads the relevant data from these computers so that she can select appropriate behaviour based on analysis of previous similar situations. This takes a bit of time, so Grandin admits that she does not work particularly well under pressure.

The brains of non-autistic people work in this way to a certain extent, but they also rely heavily on automatic responses, based perhaps on emotional reactions to what someone says or their facial expression. To help her to choose the right response, Grandin has concocted metaphors, such as visualizing relationships between people as glass doors. If you push too hard, a glass door will break; in the same way, you must often hold back and be sensitive to other people's needs if you want to get on with them. Using these metaphors, together with her mind's supercomputer filled with her observations of other people, she is able to lead a fairly normal life in what she sees as an alien world. Grandin has little sense of why other people may get upset about things to do with feelings – to her, thoughts are much more substantial and important. When the archive of the university's library was flooded, and a large number of unique, original books were ruined, she found the loss of recorded knowledge in those books painful in the same way that other people experience the loss of a friend or relative. This is not to say that people with autism are necessarily uncaring or unkind: they just need a reason to care, rather than simply feeling it.

Development in mind

The supercomputer in Temple Grandin's brain works hard to replace the automatic mind-reading ability of most people. Children who show normal development begin to acquire this ability when they are around eighteen months old. It is worth comparing the development of social skills in 'normal' children with the development of children with autism. Since the 1920s, social psychologists have carried out tests – in observation rooms with one-way mirrors, for example – to explore and document the development of social skills. It turns out that from about eighteen months old, most babies indulge in what has been called shared attention – pointing to things just to share the experience of seeing it. They spend lots of time gazing at the faces of their parents or other adults, focusing mostly on the eyes. When something unusual happens, and a child is unsure whether it is safe or dangerous, he or she refers to the adult, vying for their attention and communicating, without words: 'Look at this; is this OK?'

Simon Baron-Cohen has carried out research in this area. What he has found is that children who do not instigate social referencing or shared attention are likely to develop the symptoms of autism, normally evident around the age of three or four. Such children fix their attention more frequently on inanimate objects than on the faces of adult carers. Other studies have shown that baby boys spend less time than baby girls looking at the eyes of a carer. Another important tool in the developing social brain is pretending. From the age of about two, most children play rich, imaginative and generally participatory role-playing games, in which they might be a dragon one minute and a magician the next. Again, children with autism rarely if ever engage in such role-playing games, and girls tend to play vivid pretend games more than boys tend to do.

Also at about two or three years old, children begin to understand how other people can have feelings that are different from their own – the beginning of empathy. This is illustrated by an experiment carried out by Alison Gopnik. She presents a young child with two bowls: one with tasty crackers and one with not-so-tasty broccoli. Gopnik pretends to taste each, but demonstrates to the child that to her the crackers taste horrible and the broccoli is delicious. This she does with exaggerated gestures and facial expressions, and simple language such as 'yuk' and 'yum'. She then asks the child to choose one of the foods to give to her. Children younger than two years do not seem to take on board Gopnik's obvious feelings about each food, and nearly always offer the crackers, because they prefer them themselves. Children of two years and above do tend to offer Gopnik the broccoli, even though this is counter-intuitive since they would prefer the crackers. At this stage, it seems, children become able to understand that other people can have different views about the world from their own. A bit later on, at age five or six, children become able to understand that the same object can be interpreted in different ways. Gopnik uses ambiguous figures, such as a line drawing that could represent the head of a rabbit or the head of a duck. Children older than about six experience a switching of their interpretation of the drawing between 'duck' and 'rabbit'. Younger children – and people with autism – do not experience this switching.

One test of a child's increasing ability to 'get inside' other people's minds is the Sally-Anne Test. Originally developed by two Austrian developmental psychologists, Heinz Wimmer and Josef Perner, it was adapted by Uta Frith and her colleagues at King's College, London, for their study of the effects of autism. The test involves a scenario that is played out in front of a child, using dolls or puppets to represent the main characters. Sally has a basket, in which she keeps a marble, and Anne has a box. While Sally is out playing, Anne steals Sally's marble and puts it into her box. When asked where Sally will look for her marble when she returns, children above four years old almost always give the correct answer: in the basket where she left it, since she would be unaware that Anne had stolen it. Children younger than four tend to answer that Sally would look in Anne's box – the marble's real location – because they are unable to put themselves in Sally's position. Frith found that most children with autism – in a sample with a mental age of nine – gave the wrong answer too.

The general intelligence of people with autism – particularly those with severe symptoms – is normally lower than average. Could the fact that people with autism are not good at interpreting social cues – that they are not skilled mind readers – simply be a consequence of this lower intelligence? Two pieces of evidence suggest not: first, people with autism who do have normal intelligence, such as those with Asperger's syndrome, still have problems socializing and understanding other people's behaviour. Secondly, people with another disorder – Williams' syndrome – who also have lower than average intelligence, do have normal social skills.

Dr Helen Tager-Flusberg, a psychologist at the University of Massachusetts, is an expert in the study of children with developmental disorders, particularly problems they have in acquiring language. She has studied children with autism and those with Williams' syndrome, and has shown that children with Williams' syndrome are interested in other children, and they are very aware of when other people are happy or sad. They communicate freely and express sympathy – both happiness or sadness – about other children's feelings. They use rich and imaginative language, and take part in pretend games. Tager-Flusberg says that you see none of these behaviours in children with autism. When you give children with Williams' syndrome tasks that require them to understand what people are feeling, they do extremely well. Maude is six years old, and has Williams' syndrome. When shown a photograph of a girl being scared by a dog, she immediately gets involved with the emotions expressed in the photograph. She says that the girl is scared, because the dog is like a monster. Compare this with the way that the able children with autism had to be taught what to look out for to work out when someone looked happy. One of Tager-Flusberg's colleagues carries out a version of the Sally-Anne Test with Maude's friend Becky, another six-year-old girl with Williams' syndrome. Children with autism do not do well at this kind of test, but Becky does just fine. The experimenter shows her a crayon box, which Becky assumes contains crayons. Becky opens the box, to find that there is a sticking plaster inside. When asked what her mother would expect to be in the box if she walked in, Becky immediately answers 'crayons'. Children with autism would be likely to answer 'a sticking plaster'. Because children with Williams' syndrome are so able to carry out tasks such as these, while children with autism are particularly bad at them, Tager-Flusberg, like many psychologists, sees Williams' syndrome as the opposite of autism. The difference is in their mind-reading capabilities, their social brain.

So the deficiencies in the social brain of people with autism cannot simply be a result of lower intelligence. Instead, could they be due to damage in specific areas of the brains of these people? If so, might these areas be key parts of the social brain? In recent years, various studies have been conducted on the brains of people with autism. They have helped neuropsychologists to improve their understanding of the disorder, and have indeed provided vital clues in our quest to find the social brain.

Looking inside

Abnormalities have been found in the brains of people with autism. Some of these are found in parts of the cerebellum (the 'little brain' at the top of the brain stem) known to affect language, general cognition and attention. This might well account for some of the symptoms of autism. More relevant to our discussion of the social brain, some studies have implicated a different brain structure – the amygdalae – in the symptoms of autism. There are two amygdalae, one on either side of the brain stem. You can picture them as almond-shaped knots of nerve cells just behind your nasal cavity. These dense clumps of neurones form part of the limbic system, which is associated with emotional behaviour. The amygdalae receive signals from the eyes, nose and ears, and seem to carry out some sort of low-level, automatic computation on these signals – important in the functioning of the social brain. They also receive signals from the cortex, which carries out high-level information processing and makes associations with memories of past events. Neuroscientists have uncovered increasingly convincing evidence of the role of the amygdalae in the social brain. One way of accumulating such evidence is to use brain-scanning techniques such as MRI (magnetic resonance imaging) to investigate the activity of the amygdalae during various tasks. In 1996 Nancy Etcoff and Hans Breiter at the Massachusetts Institute of Technology did just that. The amygdalae of their experimental subjects 'lit up' on their MRI monitor screens when they showed them a series of pictures of people with fearful or threatening expressions.

The amygdalae have long been suspected to be responsible for the recognition of emotion in other people. Just how do such ideas about brain regions come about? How did neuroscientists have any idea which parts of the brain did what before the invention of MRI and other scanning techniques? There are two main ways: indirectly, by observing consistently abnormal behaviours in people or animals with damage to specific areas of their brains; and directly, by manipulating or stimulating a brain while a person or animal is conscious and recording their response or reported feelings. The amygdalae are common to many animals, including reptiles, birds and all mammals. Removal of the amygdalae in animals has been shown to reduce the animals' avoidance of strange objects, suggesting that the amygdalae are involved when we respond to fear. In several studies, mostly on rats throughout the 1980s and 1990s, Professor Joseph LeDoux of the Center for Neural Science at New York University reinforced the idea that the amygdalae are involved in an automatic response to fear. He showed that our bodies – through the amygdalae – respond to fear before we are aware of it.

Physical evidence that the amygdalae play a part in autism came in 1994 from a famous study carried out by Margaret Bauman at Harvard Medical School and Thomas Kemper at Boston University. They showed that the amygdalae of an autistic brain were smaller and more densely packed than in the normal brain. The actual neurones of the amygdalae were smaller than normal, too. In 1998 a team led by Wendy Kates of the Johns Hopkins School of Medicine in Baltimore examined the amygdalae of seven-year-old identical twin boys using an MRI scanner. One of the twins showed much more severe symptoms of autism than the other. Kates found several differences between the brains of the two boys. The hippocampus, also involved in emotional response, and the cerebellum and the caudate nucleus, involved in shifting attention from one thing to another, were all much smaller in the autistic twin's brain. So too were the amygdalae, and they were also significantly less active in the autistic twin's brain than in his brother's.

Simon Baron-Cohen and his team at the University of Cambridge have carried out similar studies. Using MRI, Baron-Cohen compared the activity of the amygdalae in people with autism to non-autistic people. Each person involved in the study was shown a series of photographs of expressive faces while their brain was scanned. Baron-Cohen's results were conclusive: people with autism do not use their amygdalae when evaluating these photographs, while others do. Again we can see that our amygdalae must be heavily involved in our social behaviour – people with autism, whose social behaviour is impaired, have deficiencies to their amygdalae. Interestingly, and perhaps not surprisingly, the brains of people with Williams' syndrome are smaller than average, but their amygdalae are the same size as in a normal brain.

Thinking it over

Just behind your forehead, above your eye sockets, lie other parts of the brain that have long been suspected to contribute to social behaviour: the orbito-frontal cortex. These sophisticated masses of neurones seem to be responsible for high-level processing of social behaviour. Our modern understanding of their function is based on evidence from case histories spanning the last 150 years. The most famous case is that of Phineas Gage, whose left orbito-frontal cortex suffered extensive damage as a result of a horrific accident in 1848. The accident happened as Gage was using an iron bar to push, or 'tamp', explosives into a hole at a construction site in Vermont. The powder exploded, firing the tamping iron out of the hole at great speed. The bar – about one metre long and six centimetres wide – shot straight through Gage's head and landed about thirty metres away. Remarkably, he survived the accident and lived for another ten years. You might imagine that such an incident would affect your behaviour: perhaps it would make you grateful to be alive. The accident did alter Gage's behaviour dramatically, but the changes were quite specific: he became irritable, bad-tempered, even rude. The accident had impaired his social brain.

Scientists at the University of Iowa have used computers to study Gage's skull which, together with the bar, has been preserved at the Harvard University Medical School Library. Using three-dimensional visualization techniques, together with knowledge of the anatomy of the brain, they have been able to work out exactly which parts of Gage's brain the iron bar destroyed. The bar passed through his chin and behind his left eye, destroying his left orbito-frontal cortex. This single case is not enough to locate the social brain – or any part of it – in the orbito-frontal region, but there have been hundreds of similar, well-documented cases. And changes in personality similar to those experienced by Phineas Gage are still occurring today – in road accident victims with severe head injury, for example. Professor Damasio, one of the team who worked on Gage's skull, says that some of his patients who have suffered severe head trauma have shown such personality changes. High-speed motorcycle crashes are perhaps the most common cause of head injury. Even though modern crash helmets are effective in dampening the force of an impact, the brain may still smash against the inside of the skull. This causes little damage to the rear of the brain, since the inside surface of the skull there is smooth. At the front, however, the inside of the skull has jagged bony ridges. When the brain hits these areas, damage is often sustained to the orbito-frontal cortex.

More evidence of the role of the orbito-frontal cortex is gleaned from a surgical procedure called lobotomy. This operation involves cutting the fibres that lead to the frontal cortex. One form of the operation was carried out by hammering an ice-pick into the brain through the orbit of the eye. Lobotomy was pioneered in 1935 by a Portuguese doctor, Antonio Egas Moniz, who called it 'leukotomy'. Between 1939 and 1950, 18,000 lobotomies were performed in the USA alone. In 1949 Egas Moniz won the Nobel Prize for medicine for his contribution, but the procedure fell out of favour during the 1950s as people began to realize that it seemed to be causing as many problems as it solved. The lives of many patients were effectively ruined after lobotomy; Egas Moniz himself was shot in the spine by one of his former patients. Often, lobotomy changed people's personalities in undesirable ways: many became unaware of other people's feelings, uninhibited, unable to conduct themselves in a civilized manner.

A little more evidence that the amygdalae and the orbito-frontal regions are major parts of the social brain is provided by the bizarre case of one of Nancy Etcoff's patients, referred to as 'LH'. In an accident, he had suffered severe damage to areas of his cortex associated with facial recognition. He cannot recognize his wife's face – she wears a ribbon that helps him identify her – or his children's faces, or even photographs of himself. He describes an experience: 'Several years ago, when I was attending a conference … I had to go to the lavatory. On the way back, I came around the corner and saw someone who I thought was a former supervisor of mine and greeted him. But there was no response. I looked again and found that I was looking at a mirrored wall, and therefore at myself.'

LH refers to himself as 'the stranger in the mirror'. But while he cannot identify faces, he can still recognize the emotions expressed by them: in other words, his social brain is intact and he can act accordingly. Neither his orbito-frontal regions nor his amygdalae were damaged in the accident. So his amygdalae continued to carry out the initial, automatic processing of signals from the senses, evaluating whether a face is sad, happy or fearful, for example, and sending the verdict to the orbito-frontal cortex. It is probably in the orbito-frontal cortex that the decision is taken on what to do with the information supplied by the amygdalae.

We have seen how this model of the social brain relates to people with autism, but can we relate it to the social behaviour of men? There is no evidence as yet in normal men of the damage to the amygdalae found in autism. Nor is there any evidence of any abnormality in the orbito-frontal cortex of men. In fact, no one has yet pinned down exactly how men's and women's social brain differs. However, one possible clue is provided through work carried out by a team led by David Skuse of the Institute of Child Health in London.

Crucial chromosomes

Skuse's study involved a rare genetic disorder called Turner's syndrome. Previous psychological studies have shown that some girls with Turner's syndrome seem to have impaired social skills. This research could point the way towards an explanation of why men are more likely to lack the social sensitivity that women seem to have. This work is highly speculative, but it could be the first step in finding the genes for social behaviour, and for understanding disorders such as autism.

It is our DNA (deoxyribonucleic acid) that determines whether we are male or female, and so consistent physical differences between men and women will be due ultimately to differences in DNA between the two sexes. The DNA is packaged as separate bundles called chromosomes, which occur in pairs, and a complete set of chromosomes is found in most cells of the body. A gene is a specific section of the DNA that makes up a chromosome. Each gene carries a coded instruction on how to build a particular type of protein. Our bodies are made mainly of proteins, so an individual's DNA in its entirety (the human genome) is like a complete build-a-human instruction manual. Under certain conditions, the various chromosomes are visible and identifiable by shape under an ordinary microscope, and their paired nature is clearly apparent. Genes on a particular chromosome correspond to the genes on the other member of the chromosome pair – although there may be many different versions of the same gene. For example, there is a gene that determines blood group, which occurs at a particular position on a particular chromosome. Each person has two versions of this gene – which may be the same or different – one on each of the two corresponding chromosomes. The blood group gene has several different forms, and the blood group of an individual will depend upon the combination of the two versions of that gene. One member of each chromosome pair comes from a person's mother and one from the father. So a person with two copies of the A version of the gene will be blood group A, while a person with one A and one B will be type AB.

A normal human being has twenty-three pairs of chromosomes, including two sex chromosomes, which may be type X or type Y. A male has an X and a Y, while a female has two Xs. Turner's syndrome – the disorder involved in Skuse's study – is caused by an irregularity in these sex chromosomes. The scientific shorthand for the chromosome complement of a normal male is 46,XY – twenty-three pairs of chromosomes, with an X and a Y for the sex chromosomes. For a female it is 46,XX. In Turner's syndrome, an individual has only one sex chromosome, an X; here, the chromosome complement is 45,X. In terms of their DNA, babies born with Turner's syndrome are neither boys nor girls. However, they grow up as girls since they do not have a Y chromosome. It is the presence of the Y chromosome that leads to the production of testosterone, which alters the usual female form of the human body, producing male body characteristics. Girls with Turner's syndrome have much in common with girls: they share the same physical characteristics (although development of their reproductive organs is impaired). However, in that they have just one

X chromosome, girls with Turner's syndrome (45,X) have something in common with boys (46,XY), too. Might they show similar traits of behaviour to boys? Can a study of the behaviour of girls with Turner's syndrome tell us anything about male-related behaviour? Skuse and his colleagues think that it can.

To what extent our DNA – our genes – determines our behaviour is an issue that has been investigated and hotly debated for as long as genes have been known to exist. This area of study, once called sociobiology, is now more often called evolutionary psychology. It is modern science's version of the age-old nature–nurture debate. Skuse and his team studied a total of eighty females, between the ages of six and twenty-five, with Turner's syndrome, administering psychological evaluations as well as carrying out genetic investigations. The psychological tests included an interview, a questionnaire and careful observation of the behaviour of the experimental subjects. The girls in the study who had social problems also reacted unfavourably to changes in routine – a behaviour commonly found in people with autism, and more often found in men than in women. Kylie, one of the girls involved in Skuse's research, was referred to him after she had shown signs of impaired social behaviour – some of the behaviours that are found in people with autism, and in typical males. If just a small part of the breakfast routine was different from normal, Kylie would react aggressively, and would be terribly confused. Her mother says that it is as if Kylie has to work through a list, that everything must be ordered. She also shows the signs of impaired social behaviour that Skuse was focusing on in his study. She has few friends, and often upsets or offends people without realizing she has done so – until she has thought it through logically, or had it explained to her in detail.

Skuse had a theory that could explain the differences between girls with Turner's syndrome who have social problems and those who do not. There are two possible sources of the single X chromosome found in a girl with Turner's syndrome: her mother or her father. All boys inherit their single X chromosome from their mother. Skuse wondered whether the females with what he refers to as 'impaired social cognition' had inherited their single X chromosome from their mother – just as boys do. Genetic tests on the sample of eighty females showed that fifty-five of them had inherited the maternal X chromosome, while the remaining twenty-five had the paternal X chromosome. What did the personality tests reveal about the social cognition of the two groups?

The results were as Skuse had suspected. He sums up: 'When we looked at those girls who had just one X chromosome, and divided them into two groups – those in whom that single X came from the mother and those in whom the single X came from the father – overwhelmingly, the social problems were in the girls whose single X came from the mother.' One illustration of this was that educational 'statementing' (identifying special needs) was three times as common in those with the maternal X chromosome than those with the paternal one.

How can we explain these findings? Skuse appeals to a relatively recent finding in genetics – that some genes are switched off on a particular member of a chromosome pair. For example, a gene on chromosome number 18 might always be inactive on the edition of that chromosome inherited from, say, the mother. This process is called imprinting: an imprinted gene is one that is deactivated. With most, non-imprinted, genes the two copies – one on each of two corresponding chromosomes – are both active. We have considered the example of the two genes that determine blood group: if a baby's mother has blood group A and the father has blood group B, then the baby will be group AB. If the gene for blood group were an imprinted one, and it was always the gene inherited from the father that was deactivated, that particular baby would have blood type A. This deactivation of a gene according to its parental origin has been found in at least twenty human genes. The process of imprinting is thought to occur when small molecules literally attach to the DNA, blocking its ability to manufacture the protein for which it holds the instructions. How does the idea of imprinted genes relate to the findings of David Skuse's research?

Skuse proposes that there might be genes found on the X chromosome that are responsible for social cognition. He thinks that the versions of these genes on the maternal chromosome are switched off – they are imprinted genes. Usually girls possess the paternal chromosome, on which the genes would remain active. Girls with Turner's syndrome who have only the paternal chromosome also benefit from those genes. However, girls with Turner's syndrome who possess only the maternal chromosome will have only switched-off copies of the genes. The maternal X chromosome is the only X chromosome that all normal males possess, so they too have only switched-off copies of the genes. Might this explain why normal males (46,XY, with X from the mother and Y from the father) and some girls with Turner's syndrome (45,X, with X from the mother) are at much greater risk of having impaired social behaviour than normal females (46,XX, with X from both the mother and father) and the other girls with Turner's syndrome (45,X, with X from the father)?

Another finding of the research was that the incidence of autism in the girls with Turner's syndrome was much higher than normal in the group with the maternal X chromosome than for normal girls or for those with only the paternal X chromosome. Again, this is true of boys, too: the occurrence of autism in males is as much as ten times as frequent as in females. Skuse's work does seem to suggest a link between our genes and our social behaviour. The social brain is almost certainly not determined by just one gene, or even many genes residing only on the X chromosome. If it did, then impairment of the social brain would be found in all males and in all of the girls with Turner's syndrome whose X chromosome came from the mother. Perhaps the social brain depends upon the collaboration of many genes, on several different chromosomes. Maybe some important ones are brought into action only when the genes on the paternal X chromosome are active – in females. Whatever genes actually are at the root of the functioning of the social brain, the situation leaves men with a much higher chance of developing autism. What possible evolutionary advantage could that bring, for it to have remained as part of our DNA?

Simon Baron-Cohen thinks he knows what the advantage of having a Y chromosome might be. He has carried out extensive psychological tests on people with autism or Asperger's syndrome and on their parents. He has carried out the same tests on a control group. The tests require very different mental skills: one involved guessing people's emotions from photographs of their eyes, the other was a visual–spatial task involving analysis of shapes. Baron-Cohen found that people with autistic-type disorders did worse than women at the first of these tasks, and so did normal men. They fared much better with the second task, however, as did normal men. The parents and grandparents on both sides of the family also did worse than the average. About five per cent of the fathers of non-autistic children are employed in some kind of engineering, compared with about twelve per cent of the fathers of children with autism. This could be explained by a bias in the brains of people with autism towards abstract, physical things and away from people, an idea that Baron-Cohen's tests seem to bear out. This would also explain why people with autism are not given to engaging with people socially. Compared with other babies, those who grow up to be autistic spend far less time looking at their parents' eyes. Similarly, boy babies spend far less time than girl babies making eye contact. Perhaps children with autism are just at one extreme of a continuum of male behaviour.

Of course, this perceived preference of males towards physical, technical things might be as much a result of socialization as the perceived superior mind-reading abilities of women. We have to exercise care in interpreting the results of studies like that carried out by David Skuse and Simon Baron-Cohen. Time and time again in the history of science, there have been examples of how the same facts can be interpreted in different ways, according to prevailing theories, religious beliefs or, of course, simply lack of enough information. For example, before the discovery of oxygen and its role in burning, most of the evidence seemed to support the prevailing idea at the time that burning involved the release of a hypothetical substance called phlogiston. Because there was no direct proof of the existence of phlogiston – only evidence that supported the idea that it existed – the theory held sway. In the same way, perhaps the conclusions of neuropsychologists will be overturned in the future, by new discoveries in genetics, physiology or psychology, or by new perspectives on existing knowledge. This does not mean that science is wrong or not worthwhile – the scientific method is a way of treading carefully along the road towards truth. But it is important to remember that our knowledge and understanding of the world are continually shifting. The results of the fascinating studies that attempt to find a link between biology and behaviour may well be interpreted in a very different way in the future. But it is also worth remembering that it was science that highlighted the fact that children with autism are not simply badly behaved because of bad parenting. And for now, current, rapidly developing theories are helping us to find the next step in the journey to find the social brain.

Social behaviour requires intelligence – a different type of intelligence from that used to take standard intelligence tests, which are the subject of the next chapter of this book.

There do seem to be fundamental differences in social intelligence between men and women, which probably do ultimately have a genetic component. Finding out how and why DNA can cause these differences might challenge some of our beliefs and our political and social values. But the real value of the quest for the social brain might be a better understanding of people with autism. Meanwhile, those lucky enough to have a fully functioning social brain can appreciate the amazing and quite automatic skills that allow human beings to be such remarkable mind readers.

NATURAL-BORN GENIUS
... the search for the nature of intelligence...

You are more intelligent than a dog, an elephant and a chimpanzee. That may be obvious, but have you ever stopped to think how amazing your intelligence is? It is easy to take for granted the incredible things that human intelligence allows us to do: read, write, explore, understand, hope, talk, make music, represent things, wonder, solve problems, work out patterns in things or the relationships between things. Parrots can speak, dogs can explore, nightingales can make music and dolphins can solve certain problems. But humans are the only animals that do all of these things, and do them well. Our minds are rich, creative, sensitive, and have given us the power to gain an understanding of the Universe around us.

It is our genes, made up of molecules of DNA, that determine our physiological characteristics and define our species. In your DNA is a complete blueprint for how to build a human body – and that includes your brain. So if there are fundamental physiological differences between humans and other animals, their origin is in DNA. Does that hold true for differences between any two human beings? It certainly does for qualities such as sex, eye colour and height. But what about behaviour and intelligence? Are some people born more intelligent than others, as a result of differences in DNA? This question is intensely controversial for many reasons, not least in terms of the lack of a precise definition of intelligence. Despite this controversy,

American behavioural geneticist Robert Plomin thinks he has found the first evidence that it is our genes that determine how intelligent we are.

Gene genius

Plomin is based at the SGDPRC (Social, Genetic and Developmental Psychiatry Research Centre), part of the Institute of Psychiatry, in London. He is one of the major figures in research into the nature of intelligence. His latest results were the culmination of six years' work, in which he followed his stern belief that there must be a genetic link to intelligence. He used the tools and procedures of molecular genetics – the study of the science of the inheritance of characteristics at the level of DNA molecules. Plomin's research was well timed: recent advances in the field of molecular genetics have made it possible actually to identify the location and functions of thousands of specific genes in plants, and in humans and other animals. In particular, a massive international effort to map out all the seventy thousand or so human genes – the Human Genome Project – is well under way. The initiative for this massive quest came from the US National Institutes of Health and the Department of Energy; in the next couple of years, the mapping process should be complete.

The human genome is the entire DNA of a human being: the twenty-three complementary pairs of chromosomes. The new genome is fixed when an egg is fertilized, defining the new individual with a complete set of forty-six chromosomes. The chromosomes present in that fertilized egg are copied to most of the cells that make up the new, growing individual. If we all have the same set of chromosomes, how can we all be different? And how can anyone assert that our DNA accounts for differences in eye colour, let alone something as subtle as intelligence? This is where genes come into the story: genes have a number of different forms. And so we are physiologically different because we have different versions of genes.

Each gene along the length of the DNA has a very specific function: it holds the instructions to produce a single protein that is used in the body. Some proteins are the building blocks of the body, including the brain; others are enzymes that regulate various functions of the body. Different versions of the same gene produce different versions of the same protein, which behave differently within the body. In some cases, this can lead to congenital diseases – for example, the inherited disease sickle-cell anaemia is the result of a particular form of the gene for the protein haemoglobin, which carries oxygen around the blood. Proteins are also important in the brain: they are the basis of many hormones and neurotransmitters, as well as being involved in the actual building of neurones. So two people with different versions of certain genes will have differences in the brain – but can those differences account for inborn differences in intelligence? Indeed, are we born with different amounts of intelligence?

Robert Plomin moved to London from Pennsylvania in 1994, the year the SGDPRC opened. The author of over two hundred scientific papers, he has a long and impressive history in the field of behavioural genetics. As long ago as 1978 he claimed to have identified a genetic basis for many behavioural aspects of laboratory animals, including learning, sexual activity, alcohol preference and aggression. In studies of twins involving humans, he also discovered evidence of a genetic component in aggression, emotional sensitivity and sociability. Unlike height or eye colour, these qualities are not easy to measure or even to define consistently and unambiguously, making any supposed genetic link difficult to prove. Intelligence suffers from the same problem, and this is one of the main reasons that his work is controversial. Nevertheless, Plomin and his colleagues set about trying to find a link, using standard intelligence tests.

Plomin considered this latest project his most challenging yet, both in scientific and political terms. It certainly has its detractors, both within the field of molecular genetics and beyond. Dr David King, editor of *GenEthics News*, a major force against Plomin's work, can see how a positive result from Plomin's work might have terrible consequences. He claims that the media would treat the results simplistically: the translation of such a finding into popular culture would be simply that those who do not have the gene for intelligence are inferior. But the over-simplification of scientific ideas could lead to more than just prejudice against individuals. Genes are the basis of race – what would it mean if it was found that certain races or ethnic groups were more likely to have the supposed 'right genes' for intelligence? David King is Jewish, and is very aware that the beliefs of the Nazis during the twentieth century were based on just this sort of premise: that breeding is everything, that we are determined purely by our genes.

As well as being challenging scientifically and politically, the possibility of a genetic basis to our intelligence is important philosophically: Plomin's work could change the way we think about human beings. It is fair to say that many academics in the field have been unwilling to believe that a genetic component exists, asserting instead that at birth we are like a blank sheet, a piece of putty to be shaped by our experiences as we develop. The question to what extent our intelligence is determined by our genes is a modern manifestation of the age-old nature versus nurture debate. Many people think that nurture builds on nature – that we are all born with about the same potential intelligence, the development of which is governed by the environment in which we grow up and the things we experience. Many scientists – even in the field of molecular genetics – saw the work as a waste of time. Plomin has always been undeterred by criticism: he sees his research as lying beyond the scope of nature–nurture debates. He thinks of it as part of a scientific quest, not a political one, to discover how the world works, and believes that the social and political consequences of any scientific discovery are the business of philosophers and politicians. This sort of argument is often used to defend research into other areas of scientific exploration, such as nuclear physics. Plomin maintains that his work really is pure science: in strict scientific terms, the funding for his project was simply to be used to search for genes that influence general intelligence.

The overall approach of Plomin's experiment was straightforward enough. He analysed specific regions of the DNA of two groups of people: one whose members had average general intelligence and one whose members had super-high intelligence. The people in the second group were each 'one in a million', as Plomin puts it. But Plomin was not actually looking for genes that create geniuses. He was searching for the first of many genes that contribute to an individual's general intelligence – the idea that underpins the work is that intelligence is a multiple-gene trait. In other words, Plomin believes that there are many genes that contribute to intelligence, at many different sites along the DNA on our chromosomes. Each gene can have many different forms. Plomin believes that some forms of each gene contribute positively, while others contribute negatively to our general intelligence.

An analogy with playing cards is useful: imagine a game where you are dealt one card from each of the four suits. In terms of this analogy the individuals with super-high intelligence in Plomin's research were each dealt a hand with four aces. A player with an average hand might have all 8s or, say, two aces and two 2s. Now imagine that there are in fact tens of thousands of different suits, and the pack consists of millions of cards. Each person is dealt a unique hand, with thousands of cards, again with one card from each suit. Suppose that only some of the many suits are important in this particular game. Then the people with the 'best' hands will have aces in most of those important suits. If you choose one of the suits important in the game, and ask each winning player to give you the card they have from that suit, most of the cards you collect will be aces. If you do the same with people who did not do so well in the game, there will be far fewer aces. If you repeat this for a suit that is not important in the game, then the likelihood is that you will have two sets of cards that you cannot tell apart. Fitting this analogy to Plomin's research, each suit is a human gene, and the face values of the cards in a particular suit are the different versions of a particular gene. So all Plomin had to do was look at the versions of particular genes in his two groups of people and determine whether a particular version occurred more frequently in the people with super-high IQ scores. With tens of thousands of genes, this is quite a task, but Plomin's previous studies had led him to a particular part of chromosome 6, which is well mapped out thanks to the Human Genome Project.

Clever Definition

Before we can begin to investigate whether or not intelligence is determined by genes, we really need to be clear about the definition of intelligence. Even here, we find controversy and disagreement. Just what is intelligence, and how can we measure it? The kind of intelligence that intelligence tests attempt to measure is called 'general intelligence'. It is supposed to be a catch-all term for cognitive ability, which is largely based on reasoning and remembering. These are vital to thought processes such as problem solving, comprehension and the use of language and mathematics, which are involved in the tasks used in standard intelligence tests. This description of intelligence may sound straightforward, but an exact definition of intelligence is almost impossible to pin down, and a reliable way to measure it is therefore just as elusive. In academic circles, the accepted meaning of the word has shifted significantly and frequently over the past hundred-odd years, and so have the theory, content and approach of intelligence tests.

The modern history of the study of intelligence begins in Victorian Britain, with Francis Galton. In 1869 Galton published his book *Hereditary Genius*, in which he set out his idea that intelligence is inborn and that some people are born with more of it than others. In that sense, Robert Plomin's research can be traced back to Galton. British naturalist Charles Darwin, who was Galton's half-cousin, was impressed by his ideas about the hereditary nature of intelligence. Darwin had previously believed that the differences in cognitive ability between any two individuals was the result of hard work alone – that people were born with almost equal potential. He was not the only one to be influenced by Galton's ideas, and Galton's methods for measuring intelligence soon became popular. In 1884 Galton set up a laboratory in South Kensington, London, where people were tested on a variety of different psychological and physiological bases, including the size of their heads and whether they could tell which of two weights was heavier. The results of these tests, Galton claimed, would give an indication of a person's general intelligence.

Galton's approach was part of an attempt to quantify everything in the natural world – biometrics – which is still a major part of scientific study. One part of Galton's biometric approach that has survived, in some academic circles at least, is the idea that intelligence is related to the speed of mental processes. Some modern intelligence theorists use reaction times or decision times as a measure of the speed with which the brain processes information, and therefore as an indication of general intelligence. The most popular test of this kind involves a box with eight lights, each with a button to press next to it. There is another button, on which you rest your hand. One of the lights illuminates, at random, and you have to react by pressing the button adjacent to that light as quickly as you can. The electronics inside the box measures how long you took to move your finger and how long it took you to move to the correct button. The test is repeated many times, so that averages of these measurements can be calculated. When compared with intelligence test scores, these measurements do correlate fairly well, and there may be some truth in them. And there are other scientists today who are continuing in Galton's tradition of measuring physical and physiological quantities to determine the nature of intelligence.

At the University of Edinburgh a differential psychologist, Ian Deary, is carrying out research into how the brain processes information, and how it relates to intelligence. He measures cranial capacity, just as Galton did, but he also uses brain scans to work out which parts of the brain are involved in the processes that give us our intelligence. This kind of research is an attempt to bridge the gap between the physiology of the brain – the hardware – and the elusive quality that we call intelligence – the software. In Deary's studies, and several others, some connection has been found between people's cranial capacities (or rather brain sizes) and the most popular measure of general intelligence, their IQs (intelligence quotients). This idea may seem crude – an elephant has a much larger brain than a human being, for example. Of course, comparing the size of the brain with body weight, humans fare better than elephants. A man's brain is slightly larger on average than a woman's, but a man's body weight is also greater on average. The value of studies into brain size and intelligence is, as yet, unknown.

Just as the roots of Plomin's work can be found in Galton's ideas, so can some of the arguments against it: Galton was the person who coined the term 'eugenics' for the idea that the human race could be bettered by 'selective breeding'. Galton was aware – or perhaps too aware – of the importance of biology and 'pedigree' in determining human traits, and proposed that careful breeding, between distinguished men and well-to-do women, would lead to a world filled with geniuses, for the good of everyone. Incidentally, this underlying concept of eugenics pre-dates Galton and the science of genetics by 2,000 years: the ancient Greek philosopher Plato put forward the idea in his great work, *The Republic*. And eugenics lived on after Galton died: it was the basis of mass sterilization programmes and propaganda in several countries that urged young people to choose someone 'fit to marry', to avoid 'pollution of the blood'.

One of Galton's claims – that a person's intelligence measured using his methods should be a predictor of his or her school or college grades – was shown to be woefully inaccurate, and Galton quickly fell out of favour. By the time he died in 1911, a new approach to intelligence – and to intelligence testing – had emerged. That new approach was pioneered by Alfred Binet, who actually died in the same year as Galton, but whose ideas dominated much of the twentieth century. Alfred Binet was a French psychologist, and impressed by Galton's attempts to use standard tests to measure differences between people. The French minister for education at the time was concerned that children with behavioural problems were receiving less teaching than their peers, because the teachers did not want to teach them. He was convinced that many of these children would therefore not reach their full potential, and ordered the creation of psychological tests to determine children's general intelligence. Binet was given the task of originating these tests, and he decided to break with the tradition of Galton and his followers. Instead of measuring what he saw as unimportant quantities, such as cranial capacity and the strength of a person's grip, Binet focused on abstract but more relevant mental processes such as judgement, comprehension, reasoning and memory. These are the same kinds of skills measured on most intelligence tests today.

But perhaps Binet's greatest contribution was the idea that we can obtain a useful measure of a person's intelligence by comparing their scores on standard tests with the average. Binet faced a fundamental problem when constructing intelligence tests for children: mental ability develops gradually over many years. The average five-year-old would not be able to solve a problem that the average ten-year-old could only just solve, for example. By giving many children of the same age a set of standard questions of varying difficulty, Binet could figure out what level of problem, say, an average seven-year-old could solve. Doing this for every chronological age would bring to light the development of the average child's mind. That is interesting in itself, but the master stroke was the idea that, by comparing a child's results with the standardized set of results, these tests could be used to compare a child's mental abilities with the average. Specifically, by comparing a child's results with the average scores for each age, you could ascertain a 'mental age' for that child. By comparing the mental age with the child's actual, chronological age, you could work out whether a child was above or below average for his or her age.

Binet's ideas were taken up by the German psychologist William Stern, who used simple mathematics to work out the 'intelligence quotient', or IQ. A simple sum is all that is needed: divide a child's mental age by his or her chronological age and multiply by 100. If a child's development exactly matches the average child for his or her age, then mental age and chronological age are the same and the calculation works out as 100 – the average IQ. If a six-year-old child is measured to have a mental age of nine according to Binet's tests, then his or her IQ is nine divided by six multiplied by 100: 150. Development of mental capability slows down dramatically as we leave childhood, so the process of estimating mental age becomes redundant in adults. But the concept of IQ – as a mathematical comparison with the average – was extended to adults. And eventually, the definition of IQ itself has shifted away from the idea of mental age. IQ is now defined using a different statistical method. Despite Binet's important contributions to the measurement of general intellectual ability, he did not really believe in the idea of general intelligence. He saw intelligence as something that pervaded all areas of mental activity, and this is why he used tests that examined skills across a wide range of mental abilities. But he believed that you could never pin down what intelligence was. To him, it was almost meaningless to say that one person was more intelligent than another.

While Binet was busy constructing his tests for French schoolchildren, a British psychologist, Charles Spearman, was setting out his ideas on what general intelligence might actually mean. Spearman's approach appealed to statistics: he was looking for correlation between test scores in several different types of ability. In other words, was a person who was good at language equally good at mathematics or remembering facts? He found that the correlation was good enough to define general intelligence, which he abbreviated to 'g'. The concept of testing people's general mental abilities was given a significant boost by the recruitment demands of World War I. The British army used psychological testing, based on Spearman's idea of g, to help them match recruits to the right jobs. The concept of general intelligence grew in popularity and, in the USA in particular, the idea of intelligence testing really took off. However, during the 1920s, rising immigration into America uncovered an inherent problem with intelligence tests: cultural bias. The tests included verbal reasoning tasks in English and visual problem solving tasks involving pictures of objects such as gramophones and tennis courts. Many of the immigrants did not speak English; some had come from places that did not have gramophones or tennis courts. The tests were clearly culturally specific and not at all relevant to these people.

Another problem associated with intelligence testing – and not unrelated to the new wave of immigration into the

USA – was the resurgence of eugenics, the idea pioneered by Francis Galton. Apart from Hitler's Germany, nowhere was the principle of eugenics applied on a larger scale than in the USA. In more than half American states during the 1920s, eugenics laws were passed that made it unlawful for certain people to marry unless they agreed to sterilization. It was appealing to some, and indeed became common, to apply labels to people according to their mental age or IQ, as defined according to Binet and Spearman. So, for example, people with IQs of over 130 were 'gifted', while those with IQs below average were labelled with varying degrees of 'retardation'. It is the latter of these two labels that was seized upon by the eugenicists of the 1920s. 'Mental retardation' was close to the term 'feeblemindedness', a label beloved of the originators of eugenics. Feeblemindedness was assumed by eugenicists to be a precursor of criminal behaviour. And when intelligence tests indicated that an adult had a mental age of twelve or below, eugenicists normally defined that person as feebleminded. Intelligence tests, then, despite their obvious cultural bias, provided some people with a seemingly objective way of showing that immigrants from Italy, Greece and countries of Eastern Europe were 'inferior'. And these were the people who were most at risk of being affected by eugenics laws. In addition, US citizens who were not immigrants but were 'mentally retarded' through, say, some congenital disorder, were often subject to the same laws. It is worth pointing out that Hitler was not in favour of intelligence testing. His eugenic theories – and eugenics in general – were based on misconceived ideas of race that went deeper than differences in intelligence.

So the concept of intelligence testing, which Binet had developed in response to a desire to provide relevant education for every child according to his or her abilities, became associated with categorizing people. School-based standardized tests became popular in many countries, including

Britain. Between the world wars, the eleven-plus examination was introduced in British schools, in order to select children who would go to grammar schools, a requirement for university entrance. After World War II, a 'tripartite system' was introduced: children went to one of three types of school, according to their ability. In addition to grammar schools, there were technical schools, which taught vocational courses, and secondary modern schools, which taught a general curriculum to a much lower level than in grammar schools.

The eleven-plus became the subject of criticism, as it seemed to determine a child's future based on a test carried out at eleven years old. During the 1950s and 1960s its use began to decline as university entrance requirements became more flexible and people began to object to the fact that standardized tests labelled children and prejudiced their educational futures. The anti-testing mood prevails to this day, as many educationists feel that such labels act as self-fulfilling prophecies. David King of *GenEthics News* says that labelling and ranking at an early age sends a signal to children perceived to have low ability along the lines of: 'Because you have a low IQ, you will be a cleaner, refuse collector or a labourer.' He sees this as a waste of people's potential – not because these jobs are unimportant, but because labelling a child at an early age narrows his or her scope in the future. King worries that if a more objective, genetic test for intelligence does result from Robert Plomin's investigations, this situation would become worse. Perhaps babies would be tested for IQ at birth … or even before?

As we have seen, the prevailing attitude of many thinkers on intelligence – that the many facets of intelligence are all manifestations of a single 'general intelligence' – had its roots in the work of Charles Spearman. There have always been those who disagree with that view, including Binet himself. During the 1980s American psychologist Howard Gardner suggested a radical approach, based on the idea that intelligence is the ability to adapt to new situations. Gardner came up with the idea of 'multiple intelligences' that widened the scope of the debate, and undermined the labelling that was the result of standardized tests of general intelligence. According to Gardner, intelligence includes linguistic, logical–mathematical, spatial, musical, bodily kinaesthetic, interpersonal and intrapersonal skills. In other words, people can be intelligent in a host of ways that help them to adapt to new situations. So an athlete who does badly on tests of intellectual ability is intelligent in a bodily kinaesthetic way. The concept of intelligence can even be extended to the social domain: people can be emotionally intelligent, for example. This view is echoed by Stephen Ceci, a psychologist at Cornell University and an expert on intelligence. He rejects the notion of IQ tests, insisting that many people with only average or below average IQs think in very complex ways. He claims that IQ measures 'school smarts' – that being a good carpenter or a good partner, for example, also requires intelligence but of a different kind. He also says that many high IQ people 'couldn't find their way out of a wet paper bag'. And yet, notwithstanding the arguments about labelling and self-fulfilling prophecy, a person's IQ does seem to correlate with their performance and their career. The average IQ of lawyers is about 128, while that of labourers is about 96. How much this correlation is due to self-fulfilling prophecy and how much to the existence of general intelligence is disputed.

Despite the approach to intelligence of people like Gardner and Ceci, and all the problems associated with IQ tests, testing remains an essential part of the education system in most countries, particularly the USA. The ETS (Educational Testing Service of America) is a huge organization. Dr Ernest Anastasia, executive vice-president of the ETS, says that the organization employs about two and a half thousand people, including a 200-strong research division. The ETS was given a national charter in 1947, and now conducts nine million tests each year. These tests, like the eleven-plus used in the UK, are an essential part of the path to a university education. For ease of marking and to avoid subjectivity, they are based on multiple-choice questions. There is a variety of tests on offer, costing between 20 and 100 dollars each, and they are marked at a rate of 8,000 per hour by an optical scanner. Many critics say that multiple-choice questions are too crude to capture something as complex as intelligence and there have been several very public attacks on the ETS. In 1980 consumer champion Ralph Nader wrote *Reign of ETS: The Corporation That Makes Up Minds*, which stimulated an outcry against the organization. Five years later, another educationist, David Owen, wrote *None of the Above*, another polemic against the ETS. This book led to the formation of an organization called FairTest, which took legal action against the ETS. In response, the ETS made changes to its methods, addressing potential test bias. But even addressing test bias does not take away the possibility of cheating, or undermining in other ways the principles of fair testing that the ETS attempts to uphold. For example, certain private organizations run courses that teach students how to increase their scores on these kind of tests. The tests are, of course, supposed to give an objective score, not just a rating on how well the students do in this sort of test. So, can an organization such as the ETS really provide information about students that could be accurate and useful?

The supporters of educational testing are very aware of the pitfalls of their testing methods, and they design tests as fairly as they can. With that in mind, many people see educational testing in the way Binet had originally devised it: as a way of providing teaching that is appropriate to each individual. This can open up new possibilities for those who have good natural ability but who may grow up in an environment that lacks intellectual stimulation. Robert Plomin himself sees the value of tests that attempt to measure natural intellectual abilities. He grew up in a large family in which educational expectations were low. It was as a direct result of educational testing that he was encouraged to attend an academic school, and therefore find his way into academia. So, for Plomin, natural-born ability is important, and tests that attempt to highlight it are certainly worth while.

Let it flow

The idea that intellectual ability is both innate and learned was an important part of the work of British psychologist Raymond Cattell. During the 1960s and 1970s, Cattell managed to find a compromise between IQ-based theories of intelligence, whose roots were in the work of Galton, and 'environmental' theories, claiming that environmental factors muddied the water too much, leaving intelligence tests measuring nothing but learned abilities and therefore inherently unfair. He agreed with Spearman's idea of g (general intelligence), but he separated it into two parts. Cattell simply formalized the existing idea that people are born with varying natural mental abilities, but their intelligence is also shaped by environmental factors, such as their schooling and their upbringing. He defined these two parts as 'fluid ability' – inborn general intelligence – and 'crystallized ability' – the result of learning. The two are clearly related: children of differing natural ability will learn different things from the same situations. This relation works in the opposite sense, too: children who grow up surrounded by books and stimulating educational experiences have a much greater chance of developing a wide range of verbal and numerical skills than those of similar ability who are starved of such experiences. These children will therefore do better on tests of crystallized ability than children of similar 'fluid' ability who do not have the same exposure to intellectual input. Tests that purport to measure fluid ability but which use questions based on verbal and numerical abilities are therefore inherently biased. Where differences in educational opportunity are related to factors such as race or economic status, the bias becomes social or cultural. This is the basis of much of the objection that has been raised to the kind of tests administered by the Educational Testing Service.

While the idea of crystallized ability might highlight bias in supposed tests of general intelligence, it can also support both the idea of g and the possibility of measuring it. In separating innate from learned abilities, Cattell presupposed that people differ in their innate ability. Assuming this is true gives credence to studies like Plomin's that attempt to investigate biological – inborn – factors in intelligence. And although tests of general ability cannot be totally free of bias, the people who design the tests are aware of the difference between fluid and crystallized ability. They make the tests as fair as they can, trying to avoid too many questions that rely on specific knowledge. Still, many popular IQ tests include general knowledge questions such as this genuine example: 'Which area of scientific study was Copernicus famous for?' (The possible answers were: 1 Biology; 2 Astronomy; 3 Chemistry; 4 Genetics.) Questions that completely eliminate this kind of specific knowledge would be abstract and perhaps difficult to understand. The closest that intelligence tests seem to come to this is the completion of series of shapes or numbers by recognizing patterns. Of course, this sort of task does improve with practice as well as with age and mental ability. However, the measurement of intelligence, along with other mental behaviours and capacities, is considered by some as an increasingly finely tuned process. Psychometric testing, as this field of endeavour is called, is sophisticated, and is becoming more and more widely used, well beyond the school environment.

In recent years, the British Army has rejected traditional interview and school examination results in favour of IQ and other state-of-the-art psychometric tests. Major Chris Allander, an army recruitment officer, reminds us that there is no army training in the school curriculum, so all new recruits must start from scratch. It is for this reason that natural cognitive abilities, and not school results, are important. The British Army is proud of the fact that this approach can offer people opportunities that they would not have otherwise had. There are many examples of recruits who have done far better in the army than their school qualifications would have allowed them to. It is worth pointing out that the questions used in the psychometric tests still rely on verbal and numerical skills, which do not necessarily reflect innate ability. To design a test that really did measure fluid ability, we would perhaps need to revert to determining reaction times or other quantities that may indicate the speed of mental processing. That explains why some researchers have tried to do just that, but the value of such research is not yet fully understood.

There are, of course, those who think that there is really no such thing as natural ability, or at least that it plays only a very minor role. One such person is Michael Howe, a psychologist at Exeter University. Howe thinks that innate ability is the wrong way to look at intelligence: that parental support is more important than natural ability, and is the key to the successful development of mental abilities. In studies of musically gifted children, he has found that parental support was a key factor: one or both parents of nearly all musically gifted children play musical instruments to a high level; music fills the house as they grow up. Michael Howe claims that experience and practice are more important than genes when it comes to intelligence. Plomin counters such arguments: when you study family members and do not take into account the genetic link, it is plausible to say that parental influence is important. But he maintains that it is also important to look at genetics: parents provide genes as well as support and experience.

Looking at the evidence

There is plenty of indirect evidence to support Plomin's view of innate mental ability. Meet Sandra Scarr, educational psychologist and expert on the influence of upbringing on children's intellectual abilities. She has visited countless schools, studying what influence the school surroundings have on children's learning and on their IQs. She is always impressed at schools that provide adequate resources and a modern curriculum, and thinks it is essential to children's development to offer as wide a range of stimulating experiences as possible. Some of the schools she visits are impoverished, with limited resources and large class sizes. At the other end of the spectrum, she sees schools that have stimulating surroundings, excellent resources and small class sizes that mean teachers can afford much more time per pupil. However, when it comes to the question of whether these factors influence IQ, she answers with a resounding 'no'.

Scarr has carried out four separate, extensive and long-term studies that have investigated possible environmental effects on IQ. In one study, she located people who had been adopted in the 1950s when they were just two months old. Scarr measured the IQs of the adoptees when they were eighteen years old. If the effects of family and schooling were important in determining IQ, then such influences would show up after the first eighteen years of life. What she found was remarkable: the IQs of the people she tested bore no relation to the IQs of the families in which they were brought up. The results could just as well have been randomly arranged. Scarr is convinced that people's genes are paramount in determining cognitive as well as other types of ability. Time and time again, while watching young children at play or engaged in educational activity, she has observed how some children naturally learn more than others. If our genes really are important in determining our intelligence, then there should be similarity between the IQs of biologically related family members. And yet different children with the same parents often have very different IQs. It is possible to explain this anomaly by returning to the analogy involving playing cards, and remembering that intelligence is assumed to be determined by a large number of genes. When a new life is conceived, two packs of cards – the genes of the mother and the father – are shuffled together. There are many different 'hands' that can be dealt from these same two packs, so it is still possible to have one child with better natural intelligence than his or her brother or sister.

But that does not really help to convince us either way – what we need to do is to compare the IQs of two individuals with exactly the same genes. Such people do exist: identical twins. However, most identical twins grow up in the same family and attend the same school, so they not only share genetic factors but environmental ones as well. Several large-scale studies of twins 'reared apart' have indicated that genes contribute at least seventy per cent to intelligence. It has been found that the similarity of identical twins' IQs seems to increase with age, suggesting that the genetic component of general intelligence is increasingly important with age, too. In one study, sixty-eight-year-old identical twins Caroline and Margaret Chang, separated at birth, had IQ test scores that were as similar to each other as the same person tested twice.

Well over one hundred studies of IQ in various contexts – twins, birth families and adoptive families – have been carried out. The most useful in helping search for a genetic basis to intelligence are the studies that involve identical twins reared apart. However, such people are rare, so most of these are of a fairly small scale. Perhaps the best-known twin studies were reported by British psychologist Cyril Burt during the 1950s. Burt claimed to have proved that intelligence is an inherited trait, based on the results of two studies of identical and non-identical twins who had been reared apart. In both studies, he arrived at a figure of 77 per cent 'heritability' – in other words, intelligence is 77 per cent genes and 23 per cent environment. In 1975, four years after his death, Burt's results were called into question. It is now largely believed that he falsified some of his data, and made up the results to match his beliefs about intelligence.

One of the largest studies ever carried out, the Minnesota Study of Twins Reared Apart, was begun in 1979 and reported its findings in 1990. The study involved more than one hundred sets of twins or triplets who had been reared apart, and put them through more than fifty hours of medical and psychological testing. The results were very similar to Cyril Burt's findings, and the Minnesota Study was certainly not faked. This does not mean that Burt's work was necessarily genuine after all, but it does suggest that genetic influence really is significant. And several other large-scale twin studies have come to the same conclusion: that inheritance – genetics – determines between 60 and 75 per cent of the intelligence of an individual.

There is generally little difference in IQ between identical twins. How does IQ vary in the population as a whole?

Scaling the heights

Intelligence – as measured in tests for g and measured as IQ (intelligence quotient) – seems to be distributed across the population in a similar way to other human attributes, such as height. A bar graph showing the heights of, say, 1,000 men at age twenty would demonstrate the distribution of heights in the population. Most men are not extremely tall or extremely short, but have heights within a range centred on the average. The bars of the graph reflect the number of men who have a particular height. Near the middle of the horizontal axis, around the average height, the bars would be tall, and near either end they would be shorter. A similar graph for 1,000 twenty-year-old women would have the same shape, but would be shifted slightly to the left since women are shorter on average than men. The profile of the graph, tracing out the tops of the bars, would look like the outline of a hill. This is called a Gaussian distribution, after the German mathematician Carl Friedrich Gauss who worked out the mathematics of this kind of curve. It is more commonly known as 'the bell curve'.

It has been found that the variation in IQ across a large, random sample of people follows the bell curve. In fact, half the people in any large, random sample will have an IQ within ten points of the average value of 100. The fraction of the population in which people have an IQ of over 130 is about 2.5 per cent. The same goes for people with an IQ of less than 70. In other words, a few people have a very low IQ, most people have an average IQ, and a few people have a very high IQ.

The fact that the distribution of IQ across any population follows the bell curve is support for the idea that intelligence is determined by many genes. To see why this is so, first consider the case of a characteristic that depends upon only one gene. A good example is the height of pea plants – in particular, the pea plants that were the subject of the first ever scientific study in genetics. During the 1860s an Austrian monk, Gregor Mendel, began a remarkable project. In an attempt to discover the rules behind the inheritance of physical characteristics, he manually fertilized over ten thousand pea plants and noted down the distributions of certain characteristics over successive generations of the plants. When he cross-bred tall plants with plants of a dwarf variety, he found that all the plants in the next generation were tall. There is a single gene that determines whether a pea plant is tall or a dwarf. A gene is a section of DNA along a chromosome found in the plants' cells, and you will remember that chromosomes occur in pairs. One member of each chromosome pair comes from each parent. So the gene that determines whether a pea plant is tall or dwarf exists twice in each plant, one copy from each parent. That gene exists in two distinct forms, which can be called T (for tall) and t (for dwarf). So any particular plant can be TT or Tt or tt, depending on which two versions of the gene it possesses. Only plants with two dwarf versions of the height gene (tt) grow up as dwarfs. Where both versions exist in the same plant, the T version 'wins' and the plant grows tall – the T version of the gene is said to be 'dominant'. This explains why the first generation of cross-bred plants were all tall: coming from parents whose height genes were TT and tt, they had to be Tt, since they received one gene from each of their parents.

What happens if you breed these first-generation plants with each other? There are four possible genetic outcomes from crossing a Tt with another Tt: TT, Tt, tT and tt. In a large sample of plants, you would expect that only one quarter of pea plants in the second generation would be dwarfs (tt). This is exactly what Mendel found. It is important to note that however many generations down the line you go, you will still only have tall and short pea plants, since the only possible combinations of T and t are TT, Tt (which is the same as tT because T is dominant) and tt. You never find pea plants with intermediate height.

The IQ of a population is not distributed in this way – only high or low – and so it is clearly not determined by a single gene. If it were, then perhaps one quarter of the population would have very low IQs (gg), while three quarters would have very high IQs (GG, Gg or gG). Could general intelligence be determined by two genes? In that case, the number of possible combinations grows from two to nine. To see how that can be so, imagine that there are two genes, A and B, which determine a particular characteristic. Assuming that each one can have two forms (A and a, B and b), then the following combinations are possible: AABB, AABb, AAbb, AaBB, AaBb, Aabb, aaBB, aaBb and aabb. With three genes, the number of different combinations is twenty-seven.

Human skin colour is thought to depend upon four genes, of which there are eighty-one different combinations. Each genetic combination produces a different concentration of melanin in the skin, and therefore a different skin colour, from pale to very dark. There is a slight natural variation in colour caused by factors such as nutrition, and so the various possible colourings merge together. People are not either black or white: the variation in skin colour in an integrated population would appear continuous. A graph of skin colour in truly integrated populations has a shape similar to the bell curve described above. With five or more genes controlling a characteristic, the variation fits the bell curve almost perfectly. Characteristics that are determined by many genes are called polygenic traits. Many examples of polygenic traits have been found, in plants, in humans and in other animals, from the colour of wheat grains to the milk yield of a large herd of cows. In each case, a graph of the variation matches the bell curve. And this is why the fact that a graph of IQ across a population follows the bell curve lends support to the idea that general intelligence is a polygenic trait. Plomin was aiming to find one of the many genes that, he believes, contribute to general intelligence.

Big news
In 1994 statistical studies of intelligence were the subject of a hugely controversial book: *The Bell Curve – Intelligence and Class Structure in American Life* by Charles Murray and Richard Herrnstein. Weighing in at a hefty 552 pages, with a further 280 pages of appendices, notes and a bibliography, it collated and interpreted the results of a large number of studies of IQ, and claimed to 'reveal the dramatic transformation that is currently in progress in American society – a process that has created a new kind of class structure led by a cognitive elite'. One of the most important studies quoted throughout the book is the National

Longitudinal Survey of Labor Market of Youth (abbreviated to NLSY). The NLSY was set up to collect information on family background, economic status and educational achievements of 12,686 Americans, all aged between fourteen and twenty-two in 1979. The survey did not originally include intelligence tests, but various psychometric tests – including IQ tests – were included from 1980 because the American Department of Defense wanted to 'renormalize' its enlistment exams. In other words, they needed the IQs of a large number of people who would be representative of the American population, so that they could adjust the scores of potential recruits based on the national average. So the IQ tests involved in the NLSY were the ones used in army enlistment. They were based on verbal and non-verbal reasoning tasks, but throughout *The Bell Curve* only one measurement – IQ as a supposed indication of general intelligence – is used consistently in the data.

Many of the findings of studies into IQ test scores presented in *The Bell Curve* were already well known – though not all undisputed – by researchers into intelligence. For example, IQ test scores seem to be rising slowly but steadily, perhaps reflecting improvements in education or health during the past century. This is why the Department of Defense wanted to renormalize their enlistment tests, which had been based on test results from enlistment during World War II. The authors divide people into five 'classes', from 'very dull' to 'very bright', based on their IQ scores. Many different aspects of American life are analysed in terms of these classes. The authors of *The Bell Curve* show that, independent of other factors, low IQ seems to increase the risk of being below the poverty line; of being on welfare; of having illegitimate children; of getting a divorce; and of being involved in crime. The evidence presented to back up these claims is impressive: there is a correlation between low IQ and each of these situations. But, as critics of the book point out, correlation is not the same as causality. In the same way, ancient Egyptians found a correlation between the appearance of certain star constellations in the night sky and the flooding of the Nile delta. These shifting constellations are not the cause of the floods, however. A correlation between low IQ and poverty might be explained in all sorts of ways, including the fact that a child growing up in poverty is not usually surrounded by an intellectually stimulating environment. Murray and Herrnstein briefly consider this idea, but conclude that 'low intelligence is a stronger precursor of poverty than low socio-economic background', and 'the traditional socio-economic analysis of the causes of poverty is inadequate and that intelligence clearly plays a role'.

The most controversial section of the book deals with IQ and race. It has apparently been shown in many reputable studies that the average IQ of people of Chinese or Japanese origin – whether in the USA or not – is higher than that of white Americans. The section of the white American population found to have the highest average IQ was made up of those people who described themselves as being of European Jewish origin. The most controversial data presented concerns black Americans (referred to in the book as African–Americans or simply 'blacks', depending on the context). Studies have consistently shown that black Americans have lower average IQs than white Americans – by as much as fifteen IQ points. This puts the average IQ of black Americans at 85.

Many questions spring to mind about this finding. For example, 'Are the differences in black and white scores attributable to cultural bias?' and 'Are the differences in black and white scores attributable to differences in socio-economic status?' and 'How do African–Americans compare with blacks in Africa on cognitive tests?' The last question is perhaps the most important one, since it would be easy for people to make the jump from 'black Americans equals low average IQ' to 'black equals low average IQ'. If the average IQ of black Americans really is lower than that of white Americans, is this because of genetic differences caused by ethnic origin – in other words, because of ancestry? Or is it because of educational disadvantages due to racist social policies? Or is it because of inherent test bias? The tests administered in the NLSY relied in part on verbal reasoning that depended on cultural reference, but several studies using tests that were supposedly culturally unbiased have also come to the general conclusion that black people's IQs are lower on average than white people's IQs. Whether these tasks were truly unbiased and objective is not certain. The tests, while supposedly culturally unbiased, still assumed a specific definition of intelligence, and still assumed that general intelligence is a meaningful concept. And even if black people in America really do have lower average IQ than white people, this could be due to environmental factors: black people in America are more likely to live in poverty than white people – and therefore less likely to grow up in an intellectually stimulating environment. And it has been found that the average IQ of black Americans is higher than that measured in black Africans. America is far richer per head than any African nation: the numbers of televisions, books and schools per thousand people are much lower in Africa than in America. Could this have something to do with the lower IQs measured? And remember – a lower IQ does not necessarily mean that you are inherently less intelligent: just that you do less well in IQ tests. In any case, you can see how this subject is a veritable minefield.

To their credit, the authors of *The Bell Curve* did embark on detailed discussions of many of the possible reasons behind their findings. But their conclusions leave a strange taste in the mouth that seems more than just having to swallow a difficult truth. At times, the language they use goes beyond pure science and into political rhetoric. Here are a couple of examples: 'The United States already has policies that inadvertently social-engineer who has babies, and it is encouraging the wrong women'; 'An immigrant population with low cognitive ability will – again, on the average – have trouble not only in finding good work but have trouble in school, at home and with the law'. Many critics objected to the book's tone and its conclusions. Charles Murray was described in an article in the *New York Times Magazine* as 'the most dangerous conservative in America'. In each of the social situations analysed in terms of IQ – such as poverty, divorce, unemployment and crime – the authors of *The Bell Curve* do consider the possible effects of environment on IQ scores. In each case, however, they remind us that most research – twin studies, for example – suggests that between 40 and 80 per cent of our intelligence is the result of our genes. The link between genes and intelligence is an important one to establish or to disprove.

We have seen that there is disagreement about whether IQ is a measure of general intelligence, and even whether the term 'general intelligence' really means anything. However, whatever it is that IQ does measure, we have seen that there is plenty of evidence that suggests that it is dependent upon genes. There are twin and adoption studies, and there is the fact that the bell curve observed with IQ is also found in many proven polygenic traits. All this evidence is important, but indirect. Robert Plomin was searching for direct evidence. He was comparing certain genes in the DNA of two distinct groups: one with super-high IQs and the other with average IQs. The group with average IQ would appear at the centre of the bell curve (at its highest point), while the second group would be out at the extreme right (near the very lowest point there). It is not too hard to find people with average intelligence, since they are the most common in the population. But how do you go about finding people with IQs of 160 or more? Where do you find one in a million? Plomin went to Iowa.

Bright sparks

Iowa State University holds an annual summer school for talented and gifted children selected, from the Midwest of the USA, for their incredible intellectual capabilities. The parents of the children come from a range of professions, and there is financial assistance for people whose parents cannot afford the fees. The summer school was founded by Camilla Benbow, an expert on gifted children, who sees it as a voyage for the mind in search of 'the least known' but 'most wondrous' knowledge, and who was also involved in the research with Plomin. During the three-week course, the teenagers study one topic in great depth. The school offers welcome intellectual challenges to people who find their normal school work easy. It also offers a chance for such people to meet others like them. This, it seems, is just as important to the children attending, since being labelled 'extremely bright' or 'gifted' can put pressure on a child.

In 1997 the course was on the subject of genetics – very fitting. One of the teachers, Jay Staker, began his preparation six months before the summer school began, and was confident of being able to deliver his part of the course. But on the first morning he was shocked by the pace at which he had delivered the material. At the end of the three weeks, he had taught the equivalent of a one-year undergraduate course in genetics.

Each of these extraordinarily intelligent children was the 'one in a million' Plomin was looking for: their genes would be studied as part of his research project. A blood sample was taken from each of them, and also – to act as an experimental control – from children with average IQ in a similar age range. A little of each of the samples was sent to two laboratories: one in Hershey, Pennsylvania, and the other in Cardiff, Wales. Both sets of samples were cultured, to produce more cells for further study, and frozen. Each new cell made in culture in the laboratory has a complete copy of the DNA of the individual from which the sample was taken.

At Hershey, in the Department of Microbiology in the College of Medicine, Pennsylvania State University, Mike and Karen Chorney, together with Nicole Seese, worked on the samples. These three researchers were aware that traditional geneticists avoided this kind of study, for two main reasons. First, as we have seen, the ethical and political issues surrounding the whole idea of a genetic link to intelligence had always steered researchers away from such a direct investigation of genes and intelligence. Second, the chance of any positive result – the discovery of a genetic link to intelligence – was perceived as minuscule. For Plomin, it is the truth that is important, not necessarily success. This research was not his first effort to find a genetic link to inheritance. Previous studies had failed to find that link and, although this was disappointing in terms of not proving his theories, Plomin's overriding emotion was relief at the avoidance of further controversy. But this latest research showed great promise for finding irrefutable evidence of that elusive first link.

The researchers at Hershey spun the blood at high speed in a centrifuge, to separate the red and white blood cells. Red blood cells are among the very few types of cells in the human body that have no nucleus, and therefore do not contain the genome. The white blood cells, on the other hand, do contain a nucleus, and the team extracted the DNA from these cells. Similar procedures were carried out in Cardiff, at the Department of Psychological Medicine at the University of Wales School of Medicine, by Mike Owens, Peter McGuffin and Johanna Daniels. Peter McGuffin has since moved to join Robert Plomin at the Institute of Psychiatry.

Both teams – in Hershey and in Cardiff – were looking for certain genetic markers. A marker is a specific section of DNA used in studies of inheritance. Proteins called restriction enzymes are used to cut the DNA, at known locations, into short pieces called restriction fragments. Markers are genes that lie near to the points at which the DNA is cut. The sizes of the fragments hold the key to which versions of genes are present in the fragments. To sort the DNA fragments, they are placed in a gel under the influence of an electrical voltage. The voltage draws them through the gel; long, heavy fragments move more slowly than short, light ones. Once this has been done for a fixed amount of time, the fragments of different lengths have been separated. By attaching a fluorescent or X-ray molecule to the DNA fragments, the positions of the fragments in the gel can be visualized. Then, the lengths of the different fragments can be worked out, along with the order of genes along the DNA. This whole process is painstaking and time-consuming, but the procedures are standard in modern genetics research. Restriction fragment length polymorphism, as this process is called, has found many applications, including DNA fingerprinting used in forensic science and paternity testing. It is also the basis of the Human Genome Project. The teams in Cardiff and Hershey were both using the technique to study genes on chromosome 6, which has been well mapped in the Human Genome Project. Specifically, the teams studied thirty-seven gene sites, looking for particular versions in the two groups. The team in Cardiff was looking at the short arm of chromosome 6, while the team in Hershey was searching the long arm. (A chromosome has a constriction along its length, called a centromere, that divides it into a 'long arm' and a 'short arm'.)

The data from Cardiff were the first to come in. Plomin and his colleague, Thalia Eley, loaded them into a computer, using statistical software to analyse the results. They began with tables showing whether a particular version of a certain gene occurred in the two groups. The results of a previous study had indicated that this gene was present more often in the group with high intelligence than in the average, control group. In this latest study, Plomin decided to double the size of the control group, to check the results. The computer quickly worked out whether a gene occurred more frequently in the high intelligence group. The results were a little disappointing: although the incidence of the gene was higher in the children with super-high intelligence, the difference was not significant enough to prove a link. And so Plomin and Eley had to wait for the next set of results, from Hershey, which looked at the long arm of chromosome 6.

When the results came in from Hershey, they were puzzling. A gene called IGF2R (insulin-like growth factor 2 receptor), was the one that Plomin and Eley were most interested in. About forty-six per cent of one group had a particular version of the gene on at least one of their two chromosome 6s, compared with 23 per cent in the other group. The results were significant, but the opposite of what Plomin had expected: it was the group with average IQs that seemed to possess the sought-for version of the gene more frequently than the group with super-high IQs. Plomin and Eley were confused by the results, and decided to re-evaluate the data the following day.

Thalia Eley came to work early the next morning, and switched on her computer, ready to begin a review of the data from the samples analysed in Hershey. She soon found that the samples had been labelled incorrectly in the computer. The set of results for the high-IQ group had been labelled as the results for the average IQ group, and vice versa. So, the results had shown a significant correlation between a particular version of the gene IGF2R and IQ after all. These results confirmed earlier suspicions about IGF2R, and provided the first hard scientific evidence of a link between IQ and our genes. Plomin estimates that this gene might cause a 2 per cent variation in IQ – about four IQ points. This may sound small, but IGF2R is probably one of many genes that influence IQ. It is not known how IGF2R, or the protein that it manufactures, might affect the brain.

There is another uncertainty: the researchers cannot even be sure that it was IGF2R that was varying between the samples. There are other, as yet unmapped, genes near to IGF2R, which would have been on the same fragments of DNA used in the restriction mapping explained above. It could be that one of these genes, and not IGF2R, is involved in intelligence. The important point is that a gene has been found that has something to do with IQ. Plomin says that people can choose to reject twin or adoption studies, but it is harder to argue with a piece of DNA.

Since the study was published in 1998, another interesting piece of evidence has arisen – this time in mice. In September 1999 a team led by Joe Tsien at Princeton University genetically engineered mice to be more intelligent. The team used a tiny glass needle to inject a gene into a fertilized mouse egg, and transferred the egg to the mother's womb. The gene the researchers inserted into the mouse genome is responsible for making a protein called NR2B. As the fertilized egg divided, to form the growing mouse foetus, the gene for NR2B was copied, along with the mouse genome, into the newly forming cells. Because it had extra copies of the gene, the mouse made more of the protein than a normal mouse. NR2B is vital in the brain, as part of a structure in neurones. Another chemical, called NDMA, which has long been associated with memory and learning, locks into particular sites on brain cells. NR2B is a vital part of those sites.

The mice with the extra gene were better at standard tasks that require intelligence, such as recognizing pieces of Lego they had seen before and learning the location of hidden platforms underwater. It seems as if the more NR2B you have, the more acute your memory. (The strain of intelligent mice was called Doogie, after *Doogie Howser, MD*, an American television series in which a boy graduates at the age of ten from Princeton University, where the research was carried out.) In the long term, this sort of research might lead to the possibility of prenatal screening of embryos to determine the likely intelligence of the baby that develops, or genetically engineering humans to be more intelligent. These possibilities are at the centre of ethical issues surrounding the work of Plomin and other molecular geneticists. If you are familiar with Aldous Huxley's futuristic fable *Brave New World*, you will remember that the population consisted of people cloned in batches, each batch having a different level of intelligence, and therefore being assigned specific roles in society. This may be a far cry from research into mouse genes, but many thinkers believe that research carried out into the genetics of intelligence could set us on a slippery slope towards something like Huxley's vision.

Sandra Scarr says that some intellectuals are fearful of the kind of research Plomin and his team are carrying out. She says that some academics propose that it should not be done or that the results should be suppressed. Scarr thinks this is unwise and patronizing to the public and the scientific community. It is better to have the information, she says: ignorance is not bliss. Camilla Benbow agrees: 'We should never be scared of knowledge.' While this may be true, what is the actual value of carrying out investigations on the influence of genes on intelligence? Benbow says that if people differ in their cognitive abilities, then knowing about the source of the differences will enable educators and politicians to respond better to them. Whether politicians and educators would respond in the best way – by providing the most nurturing and stimulating environment for every developing child according to his or her intelligence – is of course uncertain. And it is the definition and measurement of intelligence, rather than the underlying causes, that are important in providing the best possible education. Nevertheless, definite answers to the questions of whether genes determine our intelligence and how the genetic determination of intelligence works could bring new insights into our origins as a species. For example, how did intelligence develop from other animals, through evolution, and how does human intelligence differ from the intelligence of other animals? Also, discovering the link between the hardware – the physiology of the brain – and the software – intelligence – could help to treat or prevent certain brain disorders. The researchers who discovered the gene that increased the intelligence of mice have suggested that it may one day lead to drugs that could treat Alzheimer's disease or stroke.

If intelligence – and other human behaviours – is explained by biology, then philosophers may need to re-evaluate our concepts of free will and our spiritual beliefs. Plomin is more pragmatic: he says that the knowledge that intelligence is largely determined by our genes, and is only slightly influenced by our experiences, might stop over-anxious parents from flashing vocabulary cards in front of their newborn children's faces to improve their intelligence.

PHANTOM BRAINS
...the search for ghostly remains...

Driving around the S-bends on the A57 road to Blackpool, a car went out of control and left the road, hitting some trees and ending up at the bottom of a ditch. As the car stopped moving, everything went quiet. Both people in the car were alive, but in shock and had not escaped the accident unscathed. Jackie immediately realized that she had lost her left hand. An ambulance soon arrived and took Jackie and her husband to a hospital in Sheffield. Halfway there, a police car drew alongside the ambulance, and stopped it. A police officer who had recovered the hand gave it to the paramedics in the ambulance. Doctors in Sheffield worked hard to reconnect the hand, and for ten days Jackie had two hands again. But infection had set in, and began to take over; the doctors decided that the hand would have to be removed again.

This sort of experience must be traumatic and disturbing enough, but, after a few days without a left hand, Jackie began to feel something even more alarming, and for a time almost as traumatic. She felt as if she still had her missing hand. She did not like to mention this to anyone, because everyone – including Jackie – could see that there was no hand there, just a healing stump. Jackie began to doubt her sanity, because at times the hand felt as real as the one she had before the accident.

This sensation is referred to as a phantom hand. Until recently, phantom hands, arms, feet and legs – sometimes referred to as 'stump hallucinations' – were a minor scientific curiosity, but, in the last few years, scientists have begun to listen carefully to what patients say about their phantom experiences. Numerous experiments and observations in monkeys as well as in humans have provided compelling evidence that challenges existing ideas about the brain. Radical new theories have been suggested to explain the strange sensations experienced by phantom-limb patients, including the idea that the brain adjusts its internal map of the body by physically rewiring neurones in the cortex. There is an increasing number of neuroscientists actively searching for patients with phantoms, and searching too for answers.

Seeing ghosts

Digital artist Alexa Wright is a phantom hunter of a different kind. She helped to bring to light just how real a phantom can feel, working with patients such as Jackie to produce detailed pictures of what their phantoms felt like. Using digital photographs of the patients as they really were, she worked on a computer with photo-manipulation software to add in the phantoms as patients described them to her. Wright discussed the images with the patients as she was creating them, to ensure that what she captured on the computer screen – and afterwards in print – was as close as possible to a visualization of their phantom limb. In Jackie's case, the phantom that Wright visualized on the screen was about the same size as a real hand, but a bit flatter and the wrist thin and stick-like. When Jackie saw the finished image for the first time, she wept: 'When I first saw Alexa's image, I was really upset, not because I was angry about it, it was just that someone had got that image for other people to see what I feel like.'

There is tremendous variety in the images Wright has created. Phantom-limb patients often describe their arm as floating, unattached; that they can feel just a thumb attached to their stump; or that the phantom limb is stuck in a cramped and unnatural position. But the bizarre nature of these phantoms does not stop there. Patients can experience phantoms in other parts of their bodies. Patients suffering from extreme appendicitis sometimes still feel the pain after the appendix has been removed. About a third of all women who undergo mastectomy experience phantom breasts, including tingling in the phantom nipple. Some men who have their penis amputated to remove cancers have experienced phantom erections; and women have even felt phantom menstrual pains after hysterectomy.

Phantom limbs were first reported in the sixteenth century by French surgeon Ambrose Paré, who described sensations felt in absent limbs. Admiral Lord Nelson also experienced vivid phantom pain after losing his arm in an attack on Tenerife in 1797. Nelson is reported to have said that the phantom sensation gave him direct evidence of the existence of the soul. The phenomenon was first documented in detail during the American Civil War in the 1860s. American neurologist Silus Weir Mitchell wrote about the symptoms he observed in an injured soldier in a hospital in Pennsylvania. Mitchell wrote the account anonymously, and in the form of a short story, 'The Case of George Dedlow', in a popular magazine. Perhaps he did this because he was worried about what the reaction would be from the scientific community if he published them in an academic journal. The story told of how the young soldier woke up after surgeons had amputated both his legs, and asked for relief of a terrible cramp in his calf muscles. When the bedclothes were pulled back, he realized that he had no legs, let alone calf muscles.

Since the earliest accounts of phantom limbs, another phenomenon has been reported in most patients. The phantom limb can be stimulated by touching other parts of the body. Examining Jackie, neuropsychologist Peter Halligan gently touches the stump at the end of her left arm with a pen. Jackie can feel the pen touching the stump, as you would expect. But when she looks away or closes her eyes, she feels the pen touching her phantom hand. She attempts to indicate the point where she can feel the pen on her left hand, using her intact right hand. It is a point beyond the stump, in thin air. Halligan is one of the new breed of phantom hunters. Based at the Rivermead Rehabilitation Centre, Oxford, he scours the whole of Britain looking for patients who report phantom-limb symptoms. Jackie explains that inside her mind the phantom is as real as an actual hand. She was relieved to meet and talk with Halligan and Wright: at last she felt that what she was feeling was not unusual, that she was not losing her mind. In fact, some kind of phantom sensation is felt at some time by up to eighty per cent of amputees. Halligan says that he, like other neuroscientists, had tended to ignore the phenomenon of phantom limbs, treating it as a minor curiosity. 'We have neglected something that was actually telling us something about how brain processing was changing,' he says.

The sensation that a missing part of the body still exists, and the fact that this 'sensory ghost' can be stimulated by touching other parts of the body, is scientifically curious. But the story goes beyond science: into medicine. As well as just feeling that the lost limb exists, patients report feeling extreme pain in their phantom. Strong painkillers, or in some cases anticonvulsants that are normally used to treat epilepsy, do sometimes reduce the sensation, as they would do in a real limb. These phantoms exist in the mind, like hallucinations, but how and why should the brain produce such vivid and disturbing feelings? And how is it possible for normal painkilling drugs to reduce pain in part of the body that no longer exists?

When people lose someone close to them, they sometimes go through a period of denial, taking time to accept the loss; some even claim that they can still strongly feel the presence of the dead person. Could this psychological effect explain the origin of phantom limbs? Some researchers think there is a link here, while others – probably the majority – believe that the phantom-limb sensation is too vivid and too common to be explained in this way: the imaginings of a mind that cannot bear to accept the loss of part of the body cannot account for phantom sensation.

To examine the possible sources of the phantom-limb sensation, we need to know a little about what happens when something touches a real limb – one that still exists. Sensations of pressure, change in temperature and pain begin as electrical signals in nerve endings. There are two types of nerve, or neurone: sensory neurones that carry signals from around your body to your brain, and motor neurones that carry signals from your brain to your muscles. Some sensory neurones in the skin have endings that produce a signal when pressure is exerted on them, while others are sensitive to hot or cold. So when something touches the back of your hand, signals from nerve endings in your skin pass along nerve fibres that lead up the length of your arm and meet your spine at a point between your shoulders. Nerve fibres from around the body are like tributaries of a great river – the spinal cord – that flows into the brain. The adult spinal cord is normally between 40 and 50 centimetres (16–20 inches) long, and runs between your head and a point about level with your navel. However, unlike a river, the nerve pathways are not continuous. Instead, a fibre that originates in your hand terminates at the spine, passing its signals on to a different fibre in the spinal cord. So instead of water flowing into a river, you can perhaps imagine a person carrying a bucket of water: at the spinal cord, that person passes the bucket to someone else, who continues the journey. The signal passes along the second nerve fibre, up into the head, where the fibre fans out, connecting to one or more of a number of important structures.

One of these structures is the thalamus, an egg-shaped ball of neurones that acts as a relay station for nerve signals. There are two thalami, next to each other at the top of the brain stem, near the centre of the brain. Connections in the thalami transmit the nerve signals to the most sophisticated part of the brain, the cortex. Once inside the brain, nerve signals from around the body – including signals from eyes, ears, nose and mouth – are interpreted, and we have a sense of the world around us.

Mapping the body

Signals from a particular part of the body always end up in the same part of the thalamus. For this reason, there is a kind of map of the entire body within the thalamus. And in the same way, the signals from a given point in the thalamus go to a particular part of the cortex – there is a map of the body on the cortex, too. This was brought to light by remarkable work carried out in the 1950s by Canadian neurosurgeon Wilder Penfield. Working with patients who suffered from epilepsy, Penfield exposed their brains and subjected the outer cortex to low-level, localized electrical stimulation. The patients were conscious during these procedures, in order for Penfield to record their feelings as well as their actions. The point of Penfield's work was to locate the focus of epileptic seizure, but he also wanted to discover just how the brain senses the world.

He found that stimulating some areas of the cortex would produce twitches in muscles – always the same muscle for the same point on the cortex. Other areas of the cortex would bring forth vivid memories of events in the patients. Most important in our quest to discover the cause of phantom limbs, Penfield found that stimulation of certain areas in the cortex produced the sensations that seemed to come from some part of the body. By careful and systematic experimentation, he produced a detailed map of the cortex, which corresponds to sensory input from the whole body. There are actually two maps, one for each side of your body, which occur in thin strips that extend from the top of your brain down each hemisphere to points just behind your ears.

The map is distorted in two ways. In some areas of the body, nerve endings are more densely packed than in others – this means, for example, that the area of your cortex devoted to receiving sensations from your lips is larger than that receiving sensations from your upper arm. Also, parts of your body that are adjacent to each other do not necessarily appear next to each other on your cortical map. For example, your genitals are represented at the top of the map, adjacent to the representation of your feet. Similarly, your fingers are represented next to your face. Despite these distortions, the map of your body on your cortex can be represented as a little person drawn out on the surface of the brain. It has become known as Penfield's homunculus. The homunculus is clearly involved somehow in the perception of our bodies, and must also be involved in the sensation of phantom limbs. The map of the body found in the thalamus – the gateway from the spinal cord to the cortex – is also likely to be involved. But the mystery of phantom limbs – including phantom-limb pain – is far from solved.

A phenomenon related to phantom limbs is 'referred pain', where pain in internal organs is felt in (referred to) other parts of the body. So, for example, a pain originating in the heart can often be felt as pain in the wall of the chest or in the shoulders. The reason that the pain from the heart is referred to these areas in particular seems to be due to the fact that sensory neurones from the two regions enter the spinal cord at the same point. The signals originating from these two regions also arrive in adjacent areas of the cortex. The heart makes up only a tiny part of Penfield's homunculus, which explains why you are not actually very aware of your heart. The skin and muscles in the shoulder and chest wall form a larger proportion of the homunculus. It is thought that nerve signals originating in the heart 'spill over' into the area of the cortex normally involved in sensing the shoulders and chest wall. This idea is important to some of the theories that are now emerging to explain phantom limbs.

Staff and patients at the Douglas Bader Institute in Roehampton, Surrey, are familiar with phantom limbs and phantom-limb pain. The Institute specializes in making prosthetic limbs and other hardware for amputees. One of the patients, Rod, had to have the lower half of his left leg amputated after a paragliding accident. After the operation, he was relieved to have lost his leg, as up to then he had experienced intense pain. 'I was glad to lose it because the pain in the old leg was too intense, so when they took it off, my initial reaction was "great",' he recalls. 'And then the shock hit me about a week later, I suppose. The feeling of the phantom is just like permanent pins and needles. The actual pain is like a stabbing with a blunt knife.'

Phantom-limb pain can sometimes be so excruciating that patients ask doctors to try whatever they can to relieve it. Perhaps the most obvious explanation for phantom-limb pain is that nerves that were severed when the limb was amputated begin to grow back, becoming more sensitive. The severed nerve fibres that once served the amputated limb do often grow into clumps called neuromas, just inside the stump. Stimulation of the stump might produce sensations that seem to come from the lost limb because, travelling from the neuromas along the original nerve pathway, they will end up in that part of Penfield's homunculus which corresponds to the original limb. Perhaps the neuromas produce random bursts of activity, explaining why patients can feel their phantoms even when their stumps are not being touched.

There are several reasons why the explanations of phantom limbs based on stump neuromas are thought to be false. Firstly, phantom-limb pain can even be felt in limbs that are not lost. Conrad has three arms: two real and one phantom. This strange situation was the result of a motorbike accident, in which nerve fibres that connected nerve endings in Conrad's left arm to his spinal cord were ripped away. His left arm is physically still attached, however. Conrad feels intense pain in his phantom, but feels nothing from the real arm, which now dangles, paralysed. The phantom arose within a month of the accident, and Conrad describes the phantom pain in the early days: 'like your hand was being crushed and wrenched at the same time – like someone was literally trying to pull your hand out of its socket while a sixteen-ton truck is parked on it at the same time ... The pain is really in my phantom hand, not in my real hand, which is strange. You look at it, and you think, "My left hand hurts," but my left hand does nothing, it's the left hand in my head that hurts.'

As with many phantom-limb patients, pain increases in the phantom when Conrad is stressed, or if he thinks about the arm. The pain of Conrad's phantom cannot be due to a neuroma or new nerve endings in his stump: he has no stump. The case of Conrad's painful phantom, co-existing with his real arm, challenges the idea that the growth of neuromas can explain pain in a phantom in another way, too. Conrad's phantom arm is stuck in a painful, cramped position that relates directly to his accident. It is common to find that phantom limbs reflect a memory of the accident that created them, or to the pain that necessitated the removal of the real limb. In Conrad's case, the phantom hand is stuck tight as if it is gripping the handlebar of a motorcycle, and it feels as though the phantom fingers are digging into the phantom palm. Alexa Wright found this phenomenon in many of the patients with whom she worked, and has been able to visualize it in her pictures. A man who had lost his hand as a result of a firework accident, for example, felt pain emanating from the hand, as if there was an imprint of the explosion within the phantom. He asked Wright to add a red area at the centre of his hand, because he could still feel the pain of the explosion there. Some phantom-limb patients feel a watch on their wrist, a bunion on their toe or a ring on one of their fingers. These phantom memories cannot adequately be explained by the growth of neuromas or new nerve endings.

Another reason why phantom-limb pain cannot be explained as pain referred to the missing limb from new nerve endings in the stump comes from the experience of neurosurgeons, who have carried out operations to cut the nerve fibres a little further back from a stump. This isolates the newly formed neuromas from the brain, and would remove phantom sensations if they were indeed the result of neuromas. But such operations rarely have any effect on the phantom pain. Even cutting the nerves as far back as their roots in the spinal cord – an operation called a rhizotomy – normally has no effect. One theory for the cause of phantoms was that neurones in the spinal cord, starved of their normal stimulation, would produce spontaneous bursts of electrical activity. These bursts were shown to happen in certain cases, but there is plenty of evidence that it is definitely not the cause of phantom limbs. For example, phantoms experienced by patients with a complete break of the spinal cord right near the top of the spine cannot be explained by the bursting activity of neurones in the spinal cord below the break. Perhaps neuronal bursts do give rise to phantoms, but higher up – inside the head itself. One theory involved the thalamus: could bursting in the neurones of the thalamus be responsible for phantoms? Again, the answer was no. Neurosurgeons burned holes in the thalamus, with little or no effect. It is as if surgeons have chased the phantom all the way up into the brain, to the homunculus that lies on the surface of the cortex. But even removal of certain areas of the cortex has not always been successful in exorcizing the ghost of a lost limb.

Painkillers may bring some temporary relief from phantom pain. In some cases, acupuncture has also been found to ease the pain, again temporarily. A technique called TENS (transcutaneous electrical nerve stimulation) also has some benefit. In this procedure, electric voltages applied at the surface of the skin around the stump stimulate pain receptors inside the skin. Painkillers, acupuncture and TENS are effective with normal pain (in real limbs, for example). Are there any other treatments that have been effective in reducing or eliminating phantom pain in particular?

Phantom pain comes in several varieties: burning, crushing, cramps, shooting and stabbing. Phantom-limb patients normally describe one or two of these, which tend to remain the same for as long as the phantom exists. So a patient who feels only burning pain will continue to feel burning pain, and not crushing or shooting pain. This may be due to the imprinted memory of whatever led to the amputation of the real limb, as described above. However, there is evidence that each type of pain has a different cause. It has been found, for example, that burning pain is associated with a decreased blood flow in the stump, caused by a reduced temperature there. Muscles in a stump are often observed to tense up a few seconds before cramping pain, and remain tense for as long as there is pain – even though the cramp is felt in the phantom limb. More evidence for these mechanisms behind phantom pain comes from the fact that treatments to address the supposed causes do often have some effect. So ensuring good blood flow tends to reduce burning pain, while treatments that reduce muscle tone tend to reduce cramps. For burning pain, a type of biofeedback sometimes works. Patients using this technique are taught to control the temperature of their stump, at first by listening to a sound whose pitch rises and falls with temperature and then unaided.

Another, rather surprising, remedy for phantom pain involves wrapping the stump in a material, invented in

Germany during the 1960s, and now sold under the name Farabloc. The fabric is made of linen interwoven with fine steel wires. According to the manufacturer, the metal mesh shields stump neuromas from electromagnetic fields outside the body. Metal meshes like the one in Farabloc do stop electromagnetic fields, but the manufacturer's claim – that phantom limbs are caused by electromagnetic fields acting on the neuromas – does sound unlikely. However, in one strict scientific study, involving Farabloc and a similar material to act as a placebo, two-thirds of the patients involved did report some pain relief. And many users of the material do highly recommend it.

One final intriguing feature of phantom limbs is that they often shrink gradually, so that, for example, what begins as a phantom arm emanating from a stump at the shoulder slowly becomes smaller, ending up as just a finger or thumb.

Pain in the net

Ronald Melzack, professor of psychology at McGill University, Montreal, has come up with a theory to explain phantom limbs and the pain associated with them. Melzack is a world expert in phantom limbs, and has been studying them for over forty years. In the early 1990s he put forward an explanation of phantom sensations that involved a network of neurones within the brain. Because the brain is largely composed of extremely complex inter-connections of neurones, modern interpretations of many brain functions – including intelligence, memory and con-sciousness – depend on the idea of neural networks, or 'neural nets'. Melzack proposed that a sophisticated and extensive neural network, which he called the neuromatrix, produces a body image within our brains. He says that the reason why we can feel phantom sensation 'is because the neural network that makes us feel our arm as we normally feel it is the same neural network that makes us feel the phantom when we don't have the arm. The arm is gone, but the representation of that arm in the brain is still there.'

This idea incorporates the sensory map – Penfield's homunculus described above – but goes beyond it. Melzack points out that the brain does not simply react passively to sensory information, but actively creates a sense of the body, which sensory inputs from nerve endings, via the thalamus, modulate over time. This includes an input from our emotions and a sense of 'self'. These three parts – sensations, emotion and a sense of self – together create something he calls a neurosignature. So Melzack's neuromatrix – the hardware that creates the neurosignature – consists of three distinct parts working together. First, there is a sensory circuit involving the thalamus and sensory parts of the cortex. Second, he includes an emotional circuit involving the limbic system, which has long been associated with emotions. The third circuit of Melzack's neuromatrix involves the parietal lobes, one on either side of the brain. Patients who have damage to their parietal lobes seem to lose something of their concept of self. Such patients sometimes deny that parts of their bodies belong to them. The neurosignature that Melzack suggests is produced by these three circuits is a complex pattern of impulses from the neurones involved, and gives a stable impression of the complete body. Melzack uses an analogy with classical music: the neurosignature is like the theme of a piece of music, that can be played on different instruments in many different ways, but which lends stability and identity to the piece.

Melzack suggests that, because the neuromatrix is hard-wired, it must initially be determined by our genes, but that it is updated over time to incorporate changes such as chronic pain or even a wristwatch. These changes, once incorporated into the neuromatrix, and of course then into the neurosignature, would remain after the loss of a limb, explaining why amputees can still feel pains – or wrist-watches – that they had before the amputation. Support for the genetic component of the neuromatrix comes from the fact that children born with missing limbs often report phantoms. These phantoms cannot be explained by a sense of body plan that is only learned, since they have no experience of a real limb on which to draw. About twenty per cent of children born with body parts missing report phantom sensations, normally starting at about the age of five, although Melzack has heard children as young as two describe phantom limbs. Perhaps children younger than this can feel phantoms, too, but do not have adequate language to describe them or enough experience of other people to realize that they are unusual.

One of the most compelling parts of Melzack's theory is his explanation of phantom-limb pain. Melzack is particularly interested in the sensation of pain – the least well understood of the human senses. He has made several important contributions to the study of pain including co-founding, with his British colleague Patrick Wall, the 'gate-control' theory. According to this theory, pain pathways up the spinal cord can be modulated, or even blocked, by another signal entering the spinal cord, from neurones whose nerve endings are near to the ones signalling pain, or even by signals from the brain. This would explain why applying pressure, heat or electrical stimulation can help to relieve many types of pain, and why pain can often be overcome by psychological means – 'mind over matter'. Melzack believes that the neuromatrix in a person with functioning limbs would be involved in sending out signals to make the limbs move, and would also collect feedback via the senses. If a limb is missing or paralysed, the neuromatrix would send out more frequent or stronger messages, which Melzack suggests would be sensed as pain. Whatever the cause of phantom pain, Melzack thinks that the mechanisms behind it are probably the same as those behind ordinary pain, which – despite his gate-control theory – are still not well understood.

What possible explanation can there be for all the bizarre effects of phantom limbs? If one can be found, it must account for intense, imprinted pain in the phantom, which may or may not be reduced by painkillers, acupuncture or TENS. It must also account for the fact that phantom pain can be produced by physical pressure on a stump, while it can also be felt after the spinal cord has been severed (a process that would normally eliminate sensation). It must explain how a phantom limb can wither away over a long period, but rarely vanishes altogether. Finally, it must explain how the non-existent limb can be stimulated by touching different parts of a patient's body. We have seen that Penfield's homunculus plays an important role in our ability to sense the world around us, and may be at the centre of the phantom-limb phenomenon. Vital evidence in favour of this possibility came from a controversial study carried out, not on humans, but on monkeys.

Monkey business

The existence of phantom limbs seems to challenge an old assumption of neuroscience – the idea that sensations in the brain are produced only by external factors: heat and cold, pressure, light, sound. It seems that vivid sensations are created within the brain even without external stimulus. During the 1990s another cherished assumption of neuroscience was overturned, after the neural pathways in the brains of monkeys were studied. The research involved the world's most famous macaque monkeys – unwitting media superstars at the centre of an animal welfare row.

In 1981 police confiscated seventeen monkeys from a laboratory in Silver Spring, Maryland, near Washington DC. The police were called in after a volunteer working at the laboratory reported that the monkeys were being treated cruelly. The volunteer was Alex Pacheco, who the previous year had co-founded an animal rights organization called PETA (People for the Ethical Treatment of Animals), which aimed to 'establish and protect the rights of animals'. Pacheco had taken the job, at the Institute for Behavioral Research, with the intention of gathering evidence that would highlight the plight of laboratory animals. He was working for Dr Edward Taub, who together with his colleague Professor Tim Pons was carrying out research that involved cutting nerves that led from the monkeys' arms at the point at which they entered the spinal cord – dorsal rhizotomy. The researchers wanted to see whether there was any way to rehabilitate the arms.

Pacheco collected video evidence of the hardships endured by the monkeys, showing them with paralysed limbs and unbandaged wounds, living in squalor. Some of the monkeys had chewed off their fingers; their excrement filled the cages, and there was serious cockroach infestation. Pacheco took his evidence to a judge, who issued a search warrant. The police seized the monkeys, arrested Taub and collected documentary evidence from the laboratory. The case aroused widespread public interest, and people sympathetic to the monkeys' plight organized candle-lit vigils. After a long trial, Edward Taub was eventually found guilty of cruelty to animals, under the Animal Welfare Act. However, the conviction was overturned in an appeal court, on a legal technicality. The monkeys were held in captivity, but were not involved in research, for several years after they were taken from Taub's laboratory. When one of the monkeys was nearing the end of its life, in 1990, it was released back to Tim Pons (who had been cleared of all charges). Pons, and several other researchers, then followed up research that had been carried out elsewhere some years earlier.

In 1983 Dr Michael Merzenich at the University of California, San Diego, had carried out an experiment to investigate the effect on a monkey's brain of amputating its finger. Merzenich monitored the electrical activity in the monkey's cortex when he touched parts of its body.

Conventional wisdom would have predicted that the area of the cortex that corresponds to the missing finger would receive no signals, and that he would detect no signals there. However, Merzenich did record electrical activity in that area – when he touched the remaining fingers, adjacent to where the amputated one had been. So a small region of the monkey's cortex, within Penfield's homunculus, which previously received nerve signals from the finger, was now receiving signals from nerves in the adjacent fingers. The area was small – just over a millimetre square – so Merzenich did not think that new neurones had grown in the cortex to receive the signals. Instead, he reasoned that the signals were arriving at the branches of existing neurones, in the neighbouring areas of the cortex, which receive them from the unaffected fingers.

Now, in 1990, Pons and his colleagues carried out further investigations. They anaesthetized the returned Silver Spring monkey and placed electrodes on to its brain. The map on the cortex of the monkey whose finger Merzenich had amputated had undergone a small change. In Pons's version of the experiment, the neural damage was more extensive: a major nerve, from the monkey's arm, had been cut at the spinal cord. The timescale was greater, too: the nerve had actually been cut eleven years previously. So you would expect Pons and the other researchers to find reorganization on the cortex, just as Merzenich had done, but on a much larger scale. The researchers touched various parts of the monkey's anaesthetized body, and monitored the electrical activity on the cortex. To their surprise, it was touching the monkey's cheek that stimulated the area on the cortex that had once received signals from its arm. This area was about nine millimetres wide – much larger than the area affected in Merzenich's experiment. The results were repeated in tests on another seven of the monkeys. In each case, signals from the monkey's face were received across the entire area. So it seemed unlikely, if not impossible, that existing neurones were at work here. The branches of neurones in the brain do not extend far enough to explain it that way – Merzenich's explanation could not be correct.

What seems to have happened is that the neurones that once received signals from the monkey's arm atrophied, and neurones in neighbouring areas of the cortex spread to fill the space. A good way to think about what is happening when one area of the cortex map invades another is to imagine a flower bed planted with two different varieties of flower. To begin with, both varieties are healthy and they occupy separate but adjoining parts of the bed. If one variety dies off, the neighbouring plants – of the other variety – begin to spread across to the emptying patch of ground. After Pons cut the nerves that led from the monkey's arm to its brain, the area of Penfield's map that corresponded to the arm received no signals. On Penfield's map, the cheek is adjacent to the arm. So nerve signals from the cheek were ending up in the part of Penfield's map perceived as the hand as well as where they should be, in the part that corresponds to the cheek.

Neurophysiologists are uncertain to this day what causes this effect, known as cortical reorganization, but its effect on neuroscience has been dramatic. The discoveries show that the brain is flexible and adaptable, not fixed and static: it is not just the software that is changing as we go through life – the hardware rewires itself, too. Since the 1960s neuroscientists have believed that the brain is able to undergo large-scale wiring and rewiring only before birth and in the first few years of life. This explains, for example, why infants pick up languages better in their early years (and why their native tongue remains much more dominant throughout their lives).

The classic experiment that led to the view that the brain is not able to rewire itself was carried out by David Hubel and Torsten Wiesel in 1963. Hubel and Wiesel covered a new-born kitten's eye and left it covered until the kitten had developed into a mature cat. While nerve signals from the nerve endings of the body go to the area of the cortex mapped out by Wilder Penfield, signals from the eyes travel along the optic nerve to a different area – the visual cortex. Hubel and Wiesel found that the part of the cortex that would normally have received the signals from the cat's covered eye became wired to the good eye. The mapping remained the same after the cat's eye was uncovered, and the cat remained blind in one eye for the rest of its life. More importantly, when one eye of an already mature cat was covered for a significant period of time, the visual cortex underwent no changes. This is why Hubel and Wiesel concluded that the cortex is hard-wired early in life. This idea was not challenged until the experiments on monkeys carried out by Pons and his colleagues. The ability of the cortex to rewire, or at least to reorganize, which those experiments demonstrated is called 'plasticity', and it has created quite a stir in many areas of neuroscience, including the study of phantom limbs.

Primate suspect

One person who was fascinated by the consequences of plasticity and its connection with phantom limbs was Professor Vilayanur Ramachandran, professor of neuroscience at the Center for Brain Cognition at the University of California, San Diego. He was amazed to read about Tim Pons's discovery that parts of the monkey's cortex that used to receive signals from the arm was receiving them from the cheek. 'When I looked at this experiment, I nearly fell off my chair,' he says. Ramachandran wondered whether the monkey would have actually felt sensations in his non-existent, phantom hand when its cheek was stroked. It seemed natural to suggest this, since if nerve signals from the cheek were being received in the area of the cortex that normally corresponds to the hand, the monkey might feel as if its hand was being stroked. More importantly,

Ramachandran wondered whether the cortex reorganizes in the human brain in the same way as in the monkeys' brains. He suspected that it would. Humans and monkeys are quite close relatives – the anatomy and physiology of their brains are very similar, as they are both primates. Ramachandran could not really justify carrying out surgery on humans – as had been carried out on the monkeys – in order to test his theory. But he hit upon a simple and entirely non-invasive way of finding out whether there could be a connection between the brain's plasticity and phantom sensations. He found patients who had lost an arm, who had reported feeling a phantom limb. He figured that if he touched the amputees' cheeks, they might feel a sensation in their phantoms. This would prove or disprove his idea.

One of Ramachandran's patients was Derek, who had replied to a classified advert he saw in a local newspaper that called for volunteers to take part in the study. The advert was a request for amputees, and offered ten dollars per hour to those who took part. Derek, who had damaged his left arm badly in an accident six years before, wasted no time getting in touch. While he was sitting in a chair in Ramachandran's office, the professor lightly touched Derek's forehead with a pen and asked him where he had felt the pen touch. Derek replied, 'On my forehead.' When Ramachandran touched Derek's chest, Derek felt the pen touch only there. The same went for the top of his shoulder, but, when Ramachandran touched Derek's cheek, Derek could feel it touching his phantom hand as well as his cheek. Ramachandran found that the matching of touch on the face to sensation in the phantom hand was consistent – touching one part of the cheek would always trigger sensation in the middle finger, for example. Ramachandran could map out the phantom hand on Derek's cheek.

Other patients also reported feeling Ramachandran touching their cheek and their phantom hand simultaneously when he touched only their cheek, particularly when they had their eyes closed. However, Ramachandran did discover that he could also stimulate the phantom by touching the patients' arms near the shoulder. That area of the body is also represented on Penfield's map right next to the hand, on the other side from the cheek area. Again, particular locations on the shoulder always stimulated the same points on the phantom hand. So it seemed that the neurones from all around the redundant area of cortex were moving into the area that once sensed Derek's hand. Ramachandran proposed that the reorganization of the cortex was at the root of the phantom phenomenon – he calls his idea the theory of cortical remapping.

Ramachandran wondered next whether what was true of the sense of touch might also be true of the sense of whether something is hot or cold. The nerve endings that give us our sense of touch are different from those that allow us to sense heat. And the nerve pathways along which these signals travel arrive at different parts of the brain. There is a separate map of the body, in a different part of the cortex from Penfield's homunculus, which is like a temperature map of the body. Ramachandran thought that if his theory of cortical remapping could happen in Penfield's homunculus, it might happen in the temperature map too. So he dipped a cotton bud into cold water and touched Derek's face again. Derek did feel a sensation of cold in his phantom hand, and felt cold water trickling across his phantom fingers as the cold water trickled down his cheek.

To gain further evidence to support his theory, Ramachandran and some of his colleagues carried out a study using a brain-scanning technique called MEG (magnetoencephalography). This technique relies on the simple fact that electric currents produce magnetic fields. This effect is put to use in an ordinary loudspeaker: a coil of wire attached to a cone sits next to a permanent magnet. The wire carries a signal from the hi-fi amplifier – the signal is an electric current that flows backwards and forwards. The current produces a magnetic field that changes direction as the current does. This magnetic field interacts with the one produced by the permanent magnet, and the coil moves backwards and forwards making a sound. In a similar way, there are electric currents in the neurones that make up the cortex, and each one produces a tiny magnetic field. By measuring the strength of the magnetic field above particular regions of the cortex, neuroscientists using MEG can monitor which parts of the cortex are active – without opening up the skull or exposing the head to powerful X-rays. It is not possible to 'listen in' to the signals in the brain and, if it were, we would not be able to interpret what a person was thinking. However, MEG can be used to check Penfield's map, by touching various parts of the body and observing where activity is stimulated in the cortex. When Ramachandran and his colleagues used the technique to examine phantom limbs, they found that the cortex really had been remapped. On the MEG display screen, the images were clear: when the scientists touched the upper arm or the cheek of a patient who had lost a hand, the region of the cortex previously associated with the hand, as well as those associated with the cheek, became active.

Ramachandran predicted that cortical remapping would happen when other parts of the body were lost. What would happen if you lost one of your feet, for example? The feet are represented on the cortex adjacent to the area representing the genitals. So were there any people who had lost one of their feet and now felt the foot when their genitals were stimulated – during sex? Amazingly, the answer was yes. Ramachandran published his ideas in the *Proceedings of the National Academy of Science* in the USA, in 1993. Soon he was receiving phone calls from phantom-limb patients with tales to tell. And some of them had indeed felt sensations in their phantom feet while they were having sex. Some of these sensations were sexual in nature.

Ramachandran tells the story in his best-selling book, *Phantoms in the Brain* (1998). Apparently, a colleague of his suggested a different title, based on the title of another best-selling book on neuroscience, Oliver Sacks's *The Man Who Mistook His Wife for a Hat* – *The Man Who Mistook His Foot for a Penis!*

There are those who think that Ramachandran's ideas are too simplistic, but the idea of brain plasticity, at least, has become established. Other researchers have repeated his findings, and the plasticity of the brain in cats, monkeys and in human phantom-limb patients is now well documented. In some cases, reorganization of the cortex has been observed within hours of an amputation. The mechanism by which the cortical remapping takes place is still not known. There are two main theories to suggest why touching an amputee's cheek should stimulate part of the cortex normally devoted to the missing hand. First, nerves from the cheek might always have been connected to that area of the cortex. The signals entering that area from the cheek would have been inhibited before the amputation, but connections between existing neurones could strengthen when there is no input from the hand, after the amputation. This would explain why reorganization of the cortex can happen so quickly, and why some people first feel their phantoms within hours of an amputation.

The second idea is that new neurones actually grow as the existing ones die, and make new connections with other established neurones. A recent study of the brains of people who have died has brought new evidence that neurones can still grow even in older people. The patients in this well-publicized study were all suffering from terminal cancer. A chemical that is commonly used to follow the growth of cancerous cells, called Brdu (bromodeoxyuridine), was administered to the patients, to see if it might show any signs of neurone growth – molecules of this chemical attach to the DNA in dividing cells. After the patients died, their brains were examined. The researchers found Brdu in the brain – in particular in the hypothalamus – showing that new neurones had been growing there. This contrasts with the idea previously accepted, that every day from age thirty or so around 100,000 neurones die. The idea of brain plasticity has created a wave of new ideas about the brain and the suggestion of potential treatments for a range of disorders. This will be explored further in 'Lies and Delusions'.

Derek's cheek is subject to small but constant sensory input – breezes, his pulse through the blood vessels in his face, a smile. This might explain the very existence of his phantom. Some neurologists are very cautious about this explanation of phantom limbs. However, there is supporting evidence: reorganization of the cortex is definitely related to phantom pain. In 1997 Professor Niels Birbaumer and his team at the University of Tübingen temporarily eliminated phantom pain in amputees, using anaesthetics in the patients' stumps. The patients' brains were scanned before and after the anaesthetics took effect. When the patients could feel the pain, the researchers observed remapping of the cortex. But the remapping was found to be very transient: under anaesthetic it disappeared, and the cortex went back to the way it was. Another general finding of this study points to a connection between remapping and phantoms – the more extensive the remapping, the more pain is felt.

While he was working with phantom-limb patients, Professor Ramachandran was very keen to find a way to relieve phantom pain. Derek, who had participated in Ramachandran's previous studies, explained to him how, in the first two years after he lost his arm, his phantom had given him constant and terrible pain. After that, the pain had lessened a little, but when he met Ramachandran, six years after his accident, Derek still felt his phantom hand immovably cramped in an awkward position, and still painful. Ramachandran came up with another experiment that is remarkably low-tech compared with most of the techniques of modern neuroscience. He uses what he calls his mirror box, or the 'virtual reality' machine, to present phantom patients with the illusion that they have two undamaged arms.

The mirror box is constructed simply: it is made of an ordinary cardboard box with one end removed. The box sits on a table, in front of the patient, with its open end facing him or her. An ordinary mirror stands vertically down the middle, dividing the box into two chambers along its length. If the patient places one arm into the box, into one of the chambers, he or she sees a reflection of the arm, which looks as if it is in the other side of the box. The fact that our hands are symmetrical – our thumbs point towards each other when we put them face down – is important in creating the illusion that the patient has two hands. Derek was one of the first patients to try out the box. He recalls: 'The moment I put my hand in there, and saw that throbbing left phantom hand in the mirror, moving like my other hand – instantly, I felt the phantom hand move; I felt the pain withdraw a little bit; I felt the different fingers; I felt the palm; I could never move it before. I made a fist, slowly the hand started to move ... I was floored – I get teary just thinking about it.'

Ramachandran explains that after Derek had used the mirror box for about two weeks for around ten minutes every day, the phantom disappeared almost completely – all he had were the phantom fingers hanging from the shoulder. 'In a sense, we have amputated his phantom limb using a mirror,' he says. Ramachandran's explanation for this phenomenon is that perhaps the visual feedback somehow 'jump-starts' the brain so that the phantom starts moving again. In some cases, including Derek's, this can relieve the cramp in the phantom limb and ease the pain.

Ronald Melzack has tried Ramachandran's mirror box with a number of patients, and has only had one success: a patient whose phantom hand opened for the first time as a result of the procedure, and even in this case the patient's pain was not relieved. He is not convinced of the efficacy of Ramachandran's virtual-reality approach, and proposes instead that what has happened in the successful cases is due to the trust in the doctor and in medicine. In other words, Melzack thinks that there is a kind of placebo effect at work. Ramachandran admits that this could explain the effect he has witnessed with the mirror box.

Back in Oxford, Peter Halligan decided to test Ramachandran's theory and to give the mirror box a try himself. Neil is one of Halligan's patients, who has suffered extreme phantom pain since his nerves were torn in a motorbike accident. As Neil places his arms into the box, Halligan asks him whether he finds that the phantom hand opens up as he looks at the reflection of his good arm. Neil says it does: 'It seems to release the pressure of my phantom ... [reduces the pain] just like that.' The pain went from its normal seven out of ten down to essentially zero as soon as the arm was in the right position in the mirror box, and the pain came back again as soon as Neil removed his hand or closed his eyes. Whether or not the mirror box actually works, Ramachandran's theory of cortical remapping does seem to be backed up by evidence from other researchers using brain-scanning techniques, as well as by direct observation of patients. The whole idea has stimulated interest in trying out a range of new techniques to overcome phantom pain.

Opening up

Neurosurgeon Mr Tipu Aziz works at the Radcliffe Infirmary, Oxford, trying a radical and controversial approach to tackling phantom-limb pain. Wheeled into the operating theatre is Elke, ready for surgery on her exposed brain – while she is conscious. Twenty years ago, Elke was knocked down in a car accident that left her with excruciating pain in her phantom arm. Over the years doctors have tried a large number of treatments, including acupuncture and chemical and surgical nerve blockade – but all to no avail. This is why she has agreed to undergo this incredible procedure. There is no way of knowing what the long-term results might be – it is a measure of how desperate she is for relief from her phantom pain that she is willing to go through the operation.

There are no pain or touch receptors in the brain, so it is only necessary to inject local anaesthetic into the scalp. A week before the operation, under general anaesthetic, Elke's scalp was peeled back and a section of her skull 15 centimetres across was cut through in preparation for her operation. Today, Aziz staples back the scalp, and this time lifts the loosened section of skull away to reveal the brain. 'I'm just opening your skull – it might be a little uncomfortable,' he says. Once the brain is exposed, Aziz uses a small metal electrode to deliver tiny electric currents to the cortex. He needs to stimulate the cortex, just as Wilder Penfield did, in order to locate which part represents Elke's phantom arm. As the electrode becomes active, Elke reports what she feels.

At first she feels nothing, and Aziz increases the current. Suddenly, Elke's face and shoulder go into spasm – the current has caused her to have a small fit. The operation continues, with a lower current, and when Aziz locates the relevant part of the cortex he stitches the electrode in place, on to the membrane that surrounds the brain. He then attaches a wire to the electrode. The wire was previously installed underneath the skin on Elke's face, and it runs down inside her neck and to a power pack in her chest wall. The hope is that electrical pulses delivered by the power pack, arriving at the relevant spot on the cortex, will counteract the phantom-limb pain. Once everything has healed, Elke will go back to hospital and the surgeons will adjust the current from the power pack, in an attempt to change the sensation of pain to something more tolerable.

It is too soon to know whether the sort of operation that Elke endured will have the desired effect, but similar procedures are being tried elsewhere. These procedures do not only give a little hope to some patients who suffer from phantom pain, but can help neuroscientists to find out more about brain plasticity, and phantom-limb sensation in particular. In 1997 an important study that also involved 'open head' surgery was carried out by a team led by Karen Davis at the Toronto Hospital, Canada. In this case, the manipulation of the brain included subcortical structures – parts of the brain that are deeper than the cortex. The particular structure that Davis wished to investigate was the thalamus, which as we saw earlier is the relay station for nerve signals coming from the head and body. Signals relayed by the thalamus end up in the cortex, some of them contributing to Penfield's cortex map. You will remember that a sensory map of the body exists in the thalamus as well as on the cortex. A different research project, published in 1996, had shown that this map can also undergo reorganization after amputation. The role of the thalamus in the remapping could easily be forgotten, because surgery normally only exposes the cortex, and magnetoencephalography – used to investigate the remapping non-invasively – looks only at activity near to the surface, in the cortex. The electrode used in Elke's operation was more than a centimetre long and about half as wide. Davis's team used microstimulation, with much smaller electrodes, so that they could monitor and activate tiny regions of the thalamus at a time. This is necessary since the thalamus, while larger than many of the brain's structures, is still only a little more than two centimetres wide and three centimetres long.

Davis found that parts of the thalamus normally devoted to receiving nerve signals from a limb now received signals from the nerve endings in the stump. These areas of the thalamus probably still pass on the signals to the area of the cortex that represents the limb. This seems to suggest that stimulation of the stump would produce the phantom sensation – something that is quite common, though not universal, in amputees. The researchers also found that the phantom sensation could be produced by stimulating those same areas of the thalamus, when the stump was not being touched. Interestingly, the study also involved amputees who had never experienced phantoms. Stimulating the area of the thalamus corresponding to the missing limb in these patients produced no phantom sensation.

So it seems that when our brains stop receiving signals from a particular part of the body, due to amputation or to the severing of nerves, the sensory maps in our thalami and in our cortex reorganize. This probably happens through a combination of the growth of new neurones and the strengthening and weakening of the connections between existing neurones. This remapping might explain the occurrence of phantom limbs – and why touching parts of the body other than the stump, as well as in the stump itself, can produce sensations in the phantom limb. However, the cortical remapping theory alone seems to be an incomplete and inconsistent picture of how phantom limbs come to be. Not all amputees experience phantoms, for example. And in many cases, removal of the relevant part of the cortex or the thalamus does little or nothing to remove the phantom or to relieve phantom pain. Sometimes painkillers work effectively to reduce phantom pain, sometimes not. And sometimes other approaches to phantom-pain relief work in some patients, but not all. And how does cortical remapping relate to Ramachandran's mirror box – which also works in only some of the cases?

Perhaps phantom limbs can be caused by a number of different factors, some or all of which are present in a particular patient. The discovery of cortical and thalamic remapping, the plasticity of the brain, has reawakened the fascination with the way in which our brains are able to create our body image. Ramachandran says that due to plasticity, the body image is far from hard-wired, as Melzack suggests in his theory of the neuromatrix. Instead, he says it is a 'temporary construct' that the brain has created for passing our genes on to the next generation. In a sense, the whole body is a phantom that has been constructed in the brain.

Curiouser and curiouser

This fascination with the brain's creation of body image extends beyond the study of phantom limbs. Other well-documented but unexplained neurological curiosities are receiving a fresh interest since the discovery of remapping in the brain. An interesting example is a rare condition called AIWS (Alice in Wonderland syndrome), in which the sufferer's body image is severely distorted. This bewildering phenomenon is related to several different diseases. For example, an episode of AIWS normally precedes an attack of one type of migraine. There is a link, too, with glandular fever (mononucleosis). Just as Alice in the book by Lewis Carroll keeps changing size, sufferers of AIWS may feel their necks becoming longer like a giraffe's, or their whole body becoming wider. Sometimes they may feel that one half of their body is much larger than the other.

One sufferer, Lesley, explains what she commonly feels during an episode: 'I get a sensation that my hands have enlarged. They become almost as though you've put some rubber gloves on you've filled them with water and the water is expanding. And they do feel odd, the hands themselves: not only do they feel tingly, but they're huge. I feel like I could reach out and touch something a long way away. And at the same time my body is shrinking. I'm left with a feeling of only my hands – that I've gone ... that I'm reducing right down to a tiny walnut.' On other occasions, she feels herself growing taller. She feels as though she is walking on spongy, springy platform soles, and that she is looking down on everything.

AIWS was first linked to migraine in 1952, and a further link, to glandular fever, was established in 1977. But a convincing explanation for the condition has always evaded neuroscience. Brain plasticity might just be able to supply an answer. One idea is that before a migraine attack, the blood supply to the brain is disturbed, and dif ferent parts of the brain receive less blood than n Evidence in support of this comes from the exist brain of the neurotransmitter serotonin vasoconstrictor – a chemical that cause constrict, reducing blood flow. Perhaps wh body shrinking relative to her hand, the blo part of the cortex representing her hand while blood supply to the rest of the cortex is the blood supply in a particular part of the bra needed, the neurones in that part will be less short-term version of the phantom-limb ph could occur: some parts of the cortex 'take ove others. If this is true, then our body image really is just a fragile and temporary construct, and is just as plastic as the brain tha makes it.

Ronald Melzack thinks that the new theories about phantom limbs and the new approaches to treating phantom-limb pain are overly simple: 'Simple-minded approaches – like "Let's stick an electrode here and zap it or burn it out, or electrically stimulate it, or give it magnetic waves" – these are fine; give them a try, let's see what happens. But I think the real answer is going to be hard slugging down the complicated roles of endocrinology, immunology, genetics and the like.'

And Melzack is probably right. For a long time, the relationship between the wiring in our brains and our perception of our bodies and the world around us have been a question as much for philosophy as for neuroscience. And it

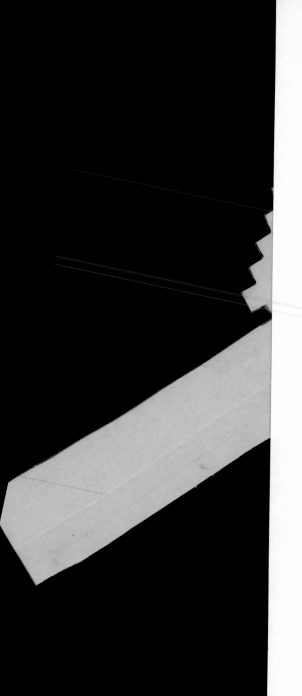

will almost certainly continue to be so for some time to come. However, the discovery of plasticity in the brain has opened up major new avenues of thought. Some of these might one day provide a more complete understanding of some of the most bizarre effects that neuroscientists and their patients have come across – including Alice in Wonderland syndrome, and perhaps phantom limbs.

LIVING DANGEROUSLY
...the search for the thrill seekers...

I t is just before dawn on a calm December morning. Elliot and John set out in a car, in pursuit of danger. They compare the excitement of what they are going to do today with that of having sex for the first time. The two thrill seekers arrive at their destination – a 200-metre-tall radio mast – while the sky is beginning to lighten, and prepare themselves. They make the slow climb up to the top of the mast, take a look out across the surrounding countryside, and jump out into the cool, calm air. As they fall, they release parachutes that will slow their descent and save their lives ... they hope. Without their parachutes, they would hit the ground at more than a hundred and fifty kilometres per hour (100 miles per hour) after just five seconds. Elliot says: 'I don't want to die, but, if that moment comes, I would deal with it. I ask myself, "Why am I doing this? Am I doing this for me?"'

Elliot and John are BASE jumping. The acronym stands for Building, Antenna, Span and Earth, and refers to the types of objects that BASE jumpers leap off. BASE jumping is illegal in most countries, although special dispensations are often made – for example, there is a 'Bridge Day' annually in the USA. There are many thousands of people involved in other dangerous sports, including high-speed downhill in-line skating, sky surfing and even canoeing down steep mountainsides. Why do these people risk their lives participating in these sports?

The world is too safe

One possible answer to the question of why people engage in extreme sports or put themselves in other dangerous situations is that the world has become too safe for them. Perhaps we humans need risk in our lives and thrive on it, and some people feel that they are not in enough danger. No one really knows how the brain goes about assessing risk, but there is evidence to support the idea that we subconsciously keep track of it. Professor Gerald Wilde of Queen's University in Ontario, Canada, has found plenty of such evidence. Wilde is an expert on risk, and in a recent study the Canadian government asked him to investigate the behaviour of drivers at railway crossings.

There are thousands of unattended level crossings, without barriers or warning lights, in Ontario. Only a handful of trains pass through them every week. The experience of Wayne, one resident of Smith Falls, Ontario, illustrates how dangerous these level crossings can be if a train arrives at just the wrong moment. For fifteen years, Wayne had travelled more or less daily over a level crossing near his home without incident. One day in 1996 he approached as normal, slowed a little as he came close to the railway lines, but kept moving. He glanced to his right as he was crossing, and saw a train hurtling towards him. The train hit his car, and turned it around. Wayne was lucky to escape with his life: 200 people have been killed crossing Ontario's level crossings during the past ten years.

Professor Wilde observed the behaviour of motorists at a level crossing over a five-week period, studying a total of 517 cars from the back of a van. As with many of the crossings, there were trees along the railway track, which obscured the motorists' view. Taking this into account, Wilde worked out at what speed motorists should approach the crossing to remain safe if a train should come. He measured the speed of each vehicle as it approached the crossing. To his surprise, he found that about seventy-five per cent of the motorists would have been hit if a train had been approaching. The fact that more people are not hit at these level crossings indicates that drivers have an awareness of the fact that trains are rare. The obvious solution, which would perhaps reduce the number of people who were not safe, was to remove the trees that were obscuring the motorists' view. Wilde and his team did just that, and Wilde recalculated the safe speed of approach given the improved view. When he observed the behaviour of drivers who now had a better view, he made a startling discovery. You would expect that the motorists, having a better view of the railway, would naturally be more safe. In fact, the effect of the improved view was that the motorists increased their speed – the level of risk stayed the same. The same effect can be seen on ordinary roads: the advent of wide, straight motorways, and safety technology such as air bags and seat belts, does not affect the level of risk of having an accident per hour spent on the road. Instead, we naturally adjust our driving to account for the risks we perceive. So, on a winding country lane in a car with no seat belts, people tend to drive more slowly and cautiously than on a motorway in a car fitted with safety equipment. It seems that this principle applies to our behaviour in general, not just to our driving.

In his book *Target Risk* (1994), Wilde documents many other examples of this phenomenon, in which people naturally and quite unconsciously maintain a certain level of risk in their lives. He calls this effect the 'risk homeostasis theory', using the term 'homeostasis' in a similar way to how French physician Claude Bernard defined it during the nineteenth century. Bernard was referring to the natural and unconscious ability of systems within the human body to maintain body temperature and chemical balances. Wilde thinks that something very similar is going on when we assess the risks of an action or activity. He defines 'target risk' as an individual's 'accepted' or 'preferred' level of risk, and explains that we seem to be happy only within a narrow window either side of this level. If the risks become too great, we will change our behaviour and take precautions to avoid undesirable outcomes. However, we also seem to adjust our behaviour if the risks become too small. He uses his theory to argue that providing technological safety measures such as seat belts, anti-lock brakes and air bags is not the most effective way to reduce the occurrence of accidents on the road. He presents plenty of convincing evidence, in addition to the study described above, that indicates that people do indeed have an awareness of how much danger they might be in, in any given situation such as driving a car.

The principle of 'risk homeostasis' sometimes stands even through dramatic changes in our way of life, such as when the motor car was invented in the late nineteenth century. Before the invention of cars, most traffic fatalities were associated with horses or horse-drawn vehicles. As car use rose during the early 1900s, so did the rate of traffic accidents associated with cars. At the same time, the rate of accidents associated with travel using horses and bicycles declined, so that per head of population, per hour of travel, the accident rate remained about the same, fluctuating slightly above and below a constant level. Wilde likens this to a thermostat, which automatically allows the temperature to drop if it is too high, and causes it to rise if it is too low. He also presents evidence that the introduction of seat-belt laws does not affect only the wearing of seat belts. The rate of accidents has been shown to rise after the introduction of such laws, again perhaps indicating that people increase their speed when they are wearing seat belts. And although people in the front seat are less likely to die in an accident if they are wearing a seat belt, the increase in the number of accidents means that the death rate remains about the same. So, if safety measures such as seat belts do not actually reduce the risks associated with driving, what is the point of introducing them?

Wilde is sure he knows the answer: 'These things are designed to improve performance, not to increase safety,' he says. 'That's why people like them.' He proposes that a person's level of target risk is determined by four factors: 'the expected benefits of comparatively risky behaviour', 'the expected costs of comparatively risky behaviour', 'the expected benefits of comparatively safe behaviour' and 'the expected costs of comparatively safe behaviour'. In the last category, he includes factors such as the discomfort and inconvenience of wearing seat belts, while in the first he includes factors such as the fact that 'making a risky manoeuvre fights boredom' – the influence of thrill-seeking behaviour.

The science of risk brings fascinating insights into human behaviour. The level of risk in an activity is directly related to the mathematical probability of the unwanted happening. Probabilities are usually given as a number between zero and one. Zero probability means that an event has no chance of happening, while a probability of one means that it definitely will. In some cases, it is easy to calculate the probability of certain events occurring. When throwing dice, for example, it has been found that the various sides of the dice land in a completely random way. This means that the probability of scoring a six on any particular die is 0.167 (one in six), since there are six faces each with an equal chance of landing face up.

We are surrounded by dangers of different types and, in many of these cases, risk cannot be calculated so easily. Risk analysts cannot rely on the mathematics of random events, like rolling dice, to calculate risks in complex, real-life situations. In these situations, risks can only be estimated using figures collected in large-scale studies or surveys across a large population and over a significant amount of time. So figures for the risk of accident per hour behind the wheel, for example, are calculated using data about the number of people driving, and the numbers of accidents that occur. Using this sort of analysis, the probability (risk) throughout a person's life of dying from a heart attack is about 0.25 (one in four), while the probability of dying as a result of being hit by lightning is about 0.00000001 (one in ten million).

Many of us are unaware of some of the very ordinary everyday risks that surround us. From the moment we wake up, being alive is dangerous. Every year in the UK, twenty people are electrocuted by their bedside lamp or alarm clock. Another twenty die as they fall getting out of bed. Thirty people die from drowning in their morning bath, and sixty are seriously injured putting on their socks. And a shocking 600 people each year die from falling down stairs – nearly two people per day. In the USA, around 6,000 people manage to injure themselves with their bedclothes. If we tried to make the world perfectly safe, we would have to remove stairs, beds and baths. Gerald Wilde puts it simply: 'Zero risk is not an option.' We can install as many safety measures as we like, and try to reduce the risks we can control (the risk of heart attack, for example), but we can never do away with risk altogether. And if we did, the world would cease to be interesting and enjoyable.

Imagining that the world can be or should be totally safe can not only make it boring – it can be dangerous. One evening in 1996 Verity and her husband were watching a *World in Action* programme about the risks to women who take contraceptive pills. The brand that Verity was taking was featured. The programme did say that the risks to women's health of taking this pill were within government limits, but it also showed the newly discovered and nasty side effects of the pill on some of the people who had suffered them. In particular, it showed women who had suffered blood clots as a result of taking the pills. The blood clots had been transported in blood vessels to the brain, where they blocked the blood supply, causing convulsions and sometimes death. Verity threw her pills into the bathroom bin the following morning, and two weeks later found out that she was pregnant. Thirty-two weeks into the pregnancy, she went for a routine check-up and was diagnosed with pre-eclampsia. This dangerous condition is one of the major risks involved in pregnancy, and is the result of a build-up of toxins in the blood. It causes high blood pressure and swelling of the hands and face; if not treated quickly and effectively, it can be fatal.

Verity was treated by consultant obstetrician Richard Johanson, who says that her kidneys were not functioning properly as result of the condition. She had an emergency caesarean section and, even after this operation, her condition did not improve for a long time: her heart could not cope, and there was a build-up of fluid in the lungs. It was a 'near miss', as Johanson puts it, and 'in times past or in other places present, she might have died'. He adds: 'Pregnancy is more of a risk than taking the pill. If half a million women who were taking Verity's pill stopped taking it, maybe one life would be saved. If half a million women became pregnant, between twenty-five and thirty would die.' There are many good arguments for and against the contraceptive pill. But in terms of risk, since the pill reduces the number of pregnancies, it reduces the risk of complications of pregnancy, such as pre-eclampsia. This applies to other methods of contraception, too, of course; but the point is that every action has a risk.

Television news programmes and the newspapers bring us horror stories every day, painting a picture of our world as a place filled with danger. We see a world in which aeroplane crashes, mass murder, rape and other violent crimes seem to be rife, and there is danger around every corner. And we see a world filled with incurable diseases, and in which the food we eat or give to our children can affect our health. In 1982, for example, there were reports of a new disease, which was spread by a virus and seemed to affect only gay men. Initially called 'gay-related immune deficiency' or GRID, it was renamed as AIDS (acquired immune deficiency syndrome) when it was realized that it did not affect only gay men – intravenous drug users, heterosexuals and even babies were also contracting this fatal disease. By 1994 AIDS was the leading cause of death among Americans aged between twenty-five and forty-four, and there was a worrying increase in the number of reported cases worldwide. AIDS was an epidemic and, due to some effective campaigning, no one was unaware of its dangers.

In 1986, this time in the UK, another health issue began to hit the headlines: it was in this year that the first case of BSE (bovine spongiform encephalopathy) was reported. BSE is sometimes called 'mad cow disease' because it affects cows' nervous systems, causing the animals to exhibit disturbing repetitive behaviours, and eventually to degenerate completely. In 1992 people began to wonder whether BSE might affect people who ate beef from cows infected with the disease. In 1993 two farmers with BSE-infected herds died of CJD (Creutzfeldt–Jakob disease), the human form of the disease. Also in 1993, the first case of CJD that proved to be the result of eating infected beef caused a media storm. A worldwide ban on British beef soon followed, and hundreds of thousands of cows were destroyed.

More recently, the public has been made aware of toxic compounds called phthalates. Investigations of these compounds have brought to light evidence that they seem to survive for longer than was thought without breaking down into harmless substances. Furthermore, they have been found in food packaging, and in foods. A study of the effects of phthalates in rats' and in human fertilization showed that fertility was reduced by an intake of some of these compounds. There was definite evidence of a reduction in size of rats' testes, for example. A further study of phthalates found them in powdered baby milk. Add to these risks the horror stories brought to us by television and the newspapers, and the aeroplane crashes that claim hundreds

of lives and it might seem that the world is more dangerous than ever, partly due to the modern technological
lifestyle we now live.

With so many dangers in the world, why would people
want to take part in dangerous sports such as BASE jumping? Perhaps the risks from AIDS, beef, baby milk, violent
crime and aeroplane crashes are not as high as we might be
led to believe. Even at the height of the AIDS epidemic, the
risk of contracting AIDS, for those not in a high-risk category
such as intravenous drug users, was less than the risk of
dying from falling out of bed. In the UK, there were between
thirty-three and eighty-one cases of CJD, and around fifteen
deaths each year between 1990 and 1998. This is one quarter of the number of people who die from drowning in their
baths. Current estimates of the risks of eating beef on the
bone suggest that one person might die as a result of eating
such beef in the next ten years. In the same period, 6,000
people will have died falling down stairs. The tests that
showed how phthalates can affect fertility involved concentrations of the compounds far higher than those found in
foods and packaging. Aeroplane crashes, while horrific for
those involved, are rare. Air travel generally carries considerably less risk than driving – the risk of dying in an
aeroplane crash over a period of one year is about
0.000002, or one in 500,000. Before the invention of motor
vehicles such as cars and trains – despite the accidents they
undoubtedly cause – travelling great distances was very
hazardous. And for every person murdered today, it is
thought that ten were murdered in the Middle Ages. The
murder rate has been halved in the past two hundred years.
Diphtheria and polio, once common life-threatening
diseases, have been all but eradicated in most countries. For
every death from an infectious disease in the twenty-first
century, there were probably at least a hundred in the
Middle Ages. So, for many of us, the world seems to be
becoming safer, not more dangerous. Of course, people in

poorer, developing countries are generally at greater risk from disease and natural disasters than people in rich, developed countries. For example, of the 33 million or so people estimated to be living with AIDS at the end of the twentieth century, the large majority were living in poorer countries, where people have far less access to new medicines, education and health-care workers.

When the media report to us the terrible consequences of eating certain foods or of travelling on aeroplanes, they tend to highlight the bad cases – safe air travel is no news. In fact, it is easy to lose sight of the benefits of technology when you are exposed only to the 'bad news'. The concept of 'benefit' is an important part of our assessment of risk. Misunderstanding the benefits of an action can be as hazardous as miscalculating the dangers. We can make mistakes when we exaggerate or underestimate the danger, or if we the ignore or magnify the benefits.

In November 1995 poisons expert Professor John Henry of St Mary's Hospital in London was contacted about the case of a girl, Leah Betts, who had become ill at a birthday party after taking an Ecstasy tablet. Leah died, and Professor Henry correctly diagnosed that the cause of death was an excessive intake of water. Ecstasy, or MDMA (3,4-methylenedioxymethamphetamine) is a hallucinogenic drug that gives people who take it feelings of euphoria. Extreme thirst is one of the side effects of the drug and, surprisingly, too much water in certain circumstances can kill you. The media interest in the case of Leah Betts was intense. Henry says that the media used him to put the 'anti-drugs' side of the Ecstasy story. And yet, he maintains that alcohol is a far more dangerous drug than Ecstasy. 'If you ask people, "Which is more dangerous, alcohol or Ecstasy?" people will immediately say "Ecstasy" – and yet we all know that alcohol presents a far greater risk,' he says. People who take the drug report significant recreational effects. That is not the same as saying that it is not dangerous. There are certainly risks associated with using the drug, perhaps some we do not know about. However, the point is that compared with alcohol, which in one way or another claims around a hundred lives every day, Ecstasy kills only a tiny number of people – no more than one person per month. In fact, since 1985, there have been fewer than a hundred Ecstasy-related deaths, while estimates of deaths related to either long-term or short-term abuse of alcohol number around thirty thousand each year.

Perhaps part of the reason we underestimate or forget the risks associated with alcohol is that they are not reported in the media. Soon after the Leah Betts case, another young person, Mark Dogget, was out for the night at a birthday party, in his local pub. It was Mark's wish to drink one whisky for every year of his life – twenty-four. He managed this, and drank a little more on top. Outside the pub, Mark vomited and fell over. He choked on his vomit and died from lack of oxygen to his brain. That evening, Mark's father Geoff received a phone call – 'The one phone call that no parent ever wants to receive' – that his child had died. Like Leah Betts, Mark Dogget died as a result of irresponsible drug use at a party. Leah Betts's story dominated the newspapers and television news for many days, while Mark's story was reported as a small item in only one national newspaper. Professor Henry says that in his hospital cases of Ecstasy toxicity are rare, but 40 per cent of emergency cases are directly related to alcohol.

We tend to ignore this huge cost of alcohol – we perceive the benefits, but not the dangers. Geoff Dogget is bemused: 'There have been situations where people are concerned about eggs, there was the BSE scare; and it's plastered all over the daily newspapers and on the television news – but one thing they don't do is mention alcohol.' Professor Henry calls this a 'national scandal'.

It seems that our concept of risk is a little distorted. Life is safer than it has ever been, and people seem obsessed with ever smaller risks. Perhaps an explanation of this is that we need risk in our lives. Gerald Wilde says there should be 'risk in your life like salt in your soup: not too much, not too little'. We have seen that we attempt to keep risk at our own acceptable or desired level. The fact that the world is actually safer than ever might explain why people go out of their way to put themselves at great risk, by participating in extreme sports. It may also explain our fascination with 'bad news': no one wants to hear how safe the world is. Similarly, we seem to have a hunger for danger in the films and television programmes we watch. The average American teenager has seen thousands of violent deaths on television or at the cinema by the age of fifteen, while most people never see one at first hand in their entire lives. Is this our way of getting our fix of the thrills of danger? If this is the case, we are still left with the question of why some people take more risks than others. The world may be more safe than ever before, and people may strive to achieve a constant level of risk, but the level of risk that is acceptable to an individual seems to differ from person to person. Just as different people like different amounts of salt in their soup, different people seek different levels of risk. However, while the taste of soup may be a matter of preference, risk-taking seems to be programmed into us, as a result of our genes or our brain biochemistry.

Seeking the thrill seekers

If we are to discover what makes people take risks, we must be able to identify risk takers. This will not only help us to 'formalize' their behaviour, but it may allow us to extend the definition of people who seek thrills and take risks, perhaps to include those who take risks without participating in dangerous sports. Only once we have a way of identifying who the risk takers are will we be able to investigate their brain and body chemistry, and their genes, and find out what gives them their drive for danger. So our quest to understand the behaviour of thrill seekers begins with an attempt to understand and categorize the personalities of these people.

Can psychologists offer us a profile of these people? Personality testing is an inexact science, despite more than a century of thought and experiment – human personality is elusive. Part of this elusiveness comes from the fact that everyone is unique, and that people change over time. People identified by one personality test as being in the same personality category might behave in very different ways from each other in some situations, and indeed might be in different categories according to a different personality test. In fact, since we are all unique, we could each be put into a different category. Personality tests can also be tautologous – in other words, they may tell you nothing that you do not already know. Organizing people into groups according to, say, the colour of their shoes, would enable you to say nothing more about each group than what colour shoes they are wearing. And so, in a personality test, you might find out nothing more than the fact that people who engage in extreme sports enjoy, well, taking part in extreme sports! The moment you make conclusions about people's personalities that go beyond the questions you ask them, those conclusions are ultimately unsupported, and are pure conjecture.

Having said this, personality tests do have their uses, and have formed the basis of scientific research into behaviour. Standard personality tests are based on theories of personality – theories about what factors influence people's feelings, thoughts and behaviour. There are many such factors, including, no doubt, genes, biochemistry of the brain, culture, childhood experiences and pure chance. It is the first two of these that we shall be examining in detail in this chapter. Is there something in the genes and the brains of thrill seekers that is different from other people's genes and brains?

The study of personality has come a long way since the ancient Greeks first attempted to explain what influences the way we think, feel and behave. Like modern neuropsychologists, the ancient Greek philosophers believed that our personalities are determined by our body chemistry. However, their ideas were a little less sophisticated than modern ones. The accepted wisdom of the ancient Greek philosophers was that personality is a direct consequence of the four humours – fluids that were thought to make up our bodies. These humours are blood, black bile, yellow bile and phlegm. Many Greek thinkers believed that blood made people enthusiastic, black bile made people melancholy, yellow bile made people angry and phlegm made people apathetic.

The history of the modern approach to personality begins with Austrian psychologist Sigmund Freud. It was Freud who set the study of personality on scientific grounds. He realized that there are hidden factors, such as innate drives and early childhood experiences, that are important in shaping our thoughts, feelings and behaviour. He believed that these can be teased out and analysed by using such techniques as free association and the interpretation of dreams. The psychoanalytic approach was extended by Swiss psychologist Carl Jung, who included a spiritual and a cultural dimension as well as attempting to classify behaviours according to four functions of the mind: sensing, feeling, thinking and intuition. He proposed that people could approach a situation in an 'introverted' or an 'extroverted' fashion, depending on whether they drew their inspiration from inside or outside themselves.

Another way of looking at personality is the behaviourist approach, pioneered by Russian psychologist Ivan Pavlov and American psychologists John Watson and Burrhus (B.F.) Skinner. According to the behaviourists, the hidden inner workings of the consciousness are not important. Instead, they believed that our behaviours, and therefore our personalities, are learned through our experiences in a manner that is understandable, objectively testable and measurable. This was an attempt to give psychology the same firm footing as other sciences. The theories of behaviourism arose through experiments, largely on animals, in which behaviours were learned, in a predictable way, through carefully controlled stimuli. Pavlov's dogs, which he taught to salivate at the sound of a dinner bell, is a famous example, but perhaps more interesting are Skinner's pigeons, which he taught to play table tennis.

Elements of both the psychoanalytic theories of Freud and Jung, and the behaviourist theories of Skinner and Watson, survive in modern approaches to personality. Modern psychology attempts to be as objective as possible, while acknowledging the fact that the human mind is extremely complex and elusive. Advances in neuroscience have begun to bridge the gap between biochemistry and behaviour, but there is still a great deal that remains unexplained. Without a complete and consistent understanding of personality or behaviour, how can we begin to categorize risk takers? If we cannot, we will be unable to compare their brain biochemistry and their genes with those of other people. Modern personality tests normally include one or both of the following components: a personality inventory and a projective test. A personality inventory is a set of questions about a person, answered by the person himself or herself, in an interview or a written questionnaire. A projective test is one with no definite answers – instead, the person being tested is asked to interpret a story or a picture. The rationale is that the person will 'project' their personality through their interpretation. The most famous example of a projective test is the Rorschach inkblot test, which involves ten abstract pictures that look like stains made by ink soaked into blotting paper.

There is a number of different approaches to testing for and categorizing people by personality type. One widely used test is the Myers-Briggs Type Indicator (MBTI). The categories defined by this test are based on a personality inventory, and have their roots in the work of Carl Jung. The questions that make up the test are based on a person's preferences in four aspects of living: how we gather information, make decisions, organize our lives and how we find 'energy' day to day. Each category has two options, each denoted by a letter. You might prefer to find energy inside (I) or outside (E) yourself; you might prefer to gather information using only your senses (S) or using your intuition (N); you might prefer to make decisions based on thought (T) or feelings (F) you might prefer to organize your life using judgement (J) or perception (P). There are sixteen combinations using these four dimensions, including ENTJ and ISFP, for example. People categorized as ENTJ are generally self-confident, with good verbal communication skills, and make good leaders, while ISFP people have a good aesthetic sense, are trusting and sensitive, and may make good artists or teachers. Since the 1970s the MBTI has been used by many organizations to help build effective teams, by identifying who has the correct personality to be a leader, who might provide the best creative input, who might be the best communicators, and so on. According to the MBTI, risk takers fall into the categories ISTP and ESTP.

Another categorization of personality – one that has become part of the language of self-help books and magazines – divides people into three types: A, B and C. Type A people are intense, driven and often uptight. Type B people are more laid-back and easy-going. Type C people are in between A and B: not too highly strung or too laid-back. Again, a personality inventory is the basis for determining whether a person is type A, B or C. In recent years, psychologists have added another – type D. Such people apparently are insecure, socially inhibited and have a negative outlook. In which of these categories do we find the risk takers? Not in any of them: in 1996 American psychologist Frank

Farley added another – type T. According to Farley, the type T personality seeks thrills, risks and arousal. Studies based on this classification have shown that people who are type T satisfy their needs in their job – as firefighters or paramedics, for example – or in other activities, such as skydiving and, yes, BASE jumping. Apparently, not all thrill seekers fulfil their desires in physical activities: many take risks in art, business or politics. Perhaps rather more destructively, some type T people also have a greater propensity towards taking drugs or drinking excessive amounts of alcohol than the general population. If Farley is correct, then, T-type people are predisposed to risk-taking behaviour, which can bring positive or negative results.

Farley drew, in part, on the work of psychologist Marvin Zuckerman, who has carried out extensive studies of personality and behaviour. Zuckerman devised a test whose aim is to find out just how risk taking an individual is. The test results are assessed along four dimensions: thrill and adventure seeking, inhibition, susceptibility to boredom and general experience seeking. Like Farley's categorization of thrill seeking, this four-dimensional approach takes into account the expression of risk-taking behaviours in art, music, sex and in social situations, as well as a propensity to take part in dangerous sports. In his book *Behavioural Expressions and Biosocial Bases of Sensation-seeking* (1994), he suggests a strong genetic component to thrill seeking. Evidence of a genetic link comes from studies of twins, which suggest that thrill seeking is a trait which is as much as sixty-nine per cent inherited. He also looks at some of the features that thrill seekers seem to have in common: they are less likely than others to suffer from stress-related disorders, for example. He investigates what biochemical mechanisms within the brain might make thrill seekers behave as they do. One biochemical that seems to be important in thrill-seeking behaviour is an enzyme known as MAO B (monoamine oxidase type B).

Another biochemical associated with thrill seeking is the neurotransmitter dopamine.

Taking a chance on MAO

The story of the role of MAO B in risk-taking behaviour begins more than twenty years ago on the prairies of mid-western Canada when a biochemist, Dr Peter Yu, embarked on an unusual experiment. At the time he was carrying out his research, MAO had already been linked to behaviour: the level of the enzyme was known to be related to mood. In particular, high levels of MAO were found in people suffering from depression. Yu decided to study the levels of MAO in the blood of the most violent criminals he could find. Near the University of Saskatoon in Saskatchewan where he works is a penitentiary for the criminally insane, and Yu tested the concentration of MAO in the blood of some of the most violent, psychopathic inmates. 'I was hoping to be able to find some biological markers for mental disorders,' he says, 'with the reason that, first, we can understand the mechanism of the disease, and, second, maybe we may be able to provide a better strategy for treatment.'

There are two forms, or isomers, of the enzyme MAO – A and B. Both isomers are found in abundance in the brain. In the rest of the body, MAO B is found in blood platelets, while MAO A is largely locked away inside organs such as the liver. Because MAO B is found in the blood, the concentration of that form of the enzyme in the body can be worked out using a simple blood test. Yu's research involved taking blood samples from the psychopaths, spinning them in a centrifuge to separate the blood cells from the platelet-containing plasma, and determining the concentration of MAO B present using radioactive molecules that bind to the enzyme. Yu took blood samples of thirty-five prisoners, and found that the levels of MAO B in their blood were much lower than in the general population. The more violent the offences they had committed, the lower the level of MAO B – as much as one-third lower in the most violent prisoners.

Yu's results have been confirmed in several more recent studies, including one in Sweden in 1997. That study found that twenty-one out of twenty-seven juvenile offenders had levels of MAO B significantly lower than the average. At the time Yu carried out his study, he was unsure how to interpret his result. 'We were very excited by these findings ... but we really didn't quite understand what that meant to us,' he explains.

Soon after Peter Yu had carried out his research, 11,000 kilometres away in Madrid clinical psychiatrist Jose Carrasco wondered whether the reduced levels of MAO B in violent criminals were related to an increased desire for risk or sensation seeking. He wondered whether the behaviour of some of his mentally ill patients might also be partly due to the same sensation seeking desire. To check the link between sensation seeking and MAO, Carrasco chose to look at the levels of MAO B in people without mental disorders or violent criminal tendencies, but who exhibited obvious risk-taking behaviour. He knew just such a group of people: matadors. Bullfighting is extremely dangerous – every year in Spain around a hundred and fifty matadors are seriously injured, and deaths are not uncommon. And yet the matadors enjoy what they do – they relish danger. One member of Carrasco's study, Fernando Gallindo, has been injured many times, including being gored in his neck and his left lung. And yet he says: 'When you are in front of the bull, and you see his eyes, and you put the bull near you – you are the centre of the world at this moment. I like risk, because behind the risk is pleasure.'

Carrasco studied seventeen bullfighters altogether. He subjected them to two tests. First, he identified how risk taking they were, according to standard personality tests including the Rorschach inkblot test, and then he tested their blood for MAO B. All the bullfighters in Carrasco's sample had lower-than-average concentrations of MAO B. Carrasco found that the bullfighters who had come out as the most risk taking on the psychological tests had the lowest concentrations of MAO B in their blood.

Back in Canada, Peter Yu decided to take the investigation into MAO B a step further. He wondered whether people who go out of their way to avoid risk might have higher than normal levels of the enzyme. At the University of Saskatoon, Nurse Judy Hawkes helps people with various phobias. Penny-Jane, one of her patients, has a range of phobias, including extreme agoraphobia, an irrational fear of open spaces, and ochlophobia, fear of crowds. In fact, her anxiety is so pervasive that she has been diagnosed with panic disorder, in which breathlessness, faintness and palpitations are common and may happen suddenly and unpredictably even in everyday situations. She feels at ease only in her home or in her car. She has not visited the local supermarket for more than six years. For her, everyday life is full of unacceptable risks. She says that she is terrified of going into shops and that she feels 'very trapped, like an escape feeling, like I want to get out; as if there was a fire – I feel that same feeling'.

Under the care of Nurse Judy Hawkes, Penny-Jane practises overcoming her fears. At the supermarket, Penny-Jane ventures inside while Hawkes remains outside in the car park. The two speak to each other on mobile phones, so that Hawkes can monitor Penny-Jane's progress and reassure her if she becomes anxious. After just a few minutes inside the shop Penny-Jane, breathing heavily and feeling numb, can take it no more, and asks the nurse to come and rescue her. What would the levels of MAO B be like in the blood of people like Penny-Jane?

Peter Yu carried out the same test on Penny-Jane – and another twenty-eight people with a similar panic disorder – as he had done on the violent inmates of the nearby penitentiary. As he predicted, the MAO B concentration in the blood of these people was significantly higher than average. Phobias have always been assumed to originate in traumatic events during early childhood – and no doubt many specific ones do. However, here was a biochemical basis for general fearful anxiety, seemingly caused by an excess of the same biochemical as, when in lower concentrations, seemed to be responsible for the risk-taking behaviour of the violent criminals and the matadors. Moreover, since the studies of Yu and Carrasco, other studies have shown that men generally have lower levels of MAO B, which correlates with the fact that there are more risk-taking men, involved in dangerous sports or violent crime, than women. It has also been found that the levels of MAO B generally increase with age, perhaps explaining why people seem to become more cautious and less risk taking as they grow older. There seems to be a link between MAO and risk-taking behaviour. To explain what neuroscientists think that link is, we need to understand the function of MAO in the brain.

Chemicals in the brain

The two forms of MAO (monoamine oxidase) are part of a complex cocktail of biochemicals in our brains. Their job is to break down neurotransmitters – chemicals that play a vital role in the transmission of nerve signals between neurones. A neurone is surrounded by a thin membrane, and is made up of the cell body, a fibre called an axon that carries 'output' signals, and thinner fibres called dendrites, which carry 'input' signals. A neurone is subject to the inputs of hundreds or thousands of dendrites together – each one the signal from a different neurone. It is as if each one is registering a vote – the result of all the votes is either the neurone 'firing' or remaining silent. When a neurone does fire, the signal passes along the length of the axon, and neurotransmitters are released through the cell membrane at the many ends of the axon. The neurotransmitters burst forth from the end of the axon, and attach themselves to the end of a dendrite of another neurone sitting very close by. As they do, they may cause holes to open in the membrane of the second neurone. Positively charged sodium or calcium ions flood in through these holes, initiating another nerve impulse in the second neurone. The gap between one of the ends of an axon and the end of one of the dendrites of another neurone is called a synapse.

It may seem unnecessarily complicated to have this indirect transmission of nerve signals involving neuro-transmitters across a synaptic gap – why not just have the nerves connected together directly? There are in fact several reasons why it is important that the neurones do not connect directly to each other, but instead form synapses. One of them is that neurotransmitters may be either 'exci-tory' or 'inhibitory'. In other words, a signal received at some synapses will give a 'no' vote and at others, it will be a 'yes' vote. This gives the whole system a much greater flexibility. Also, the cocktail of neurochemicals in the synaptic gap can change according to mood, and this results in changes in the transmission of nerve impulses across the synapse.

There are many different neurotransmitters, each one concentrated in particular areas of the brain. For example, dopamine (hydroxytyramine) acts as both an inhibitory and an excitory neurotransmitter, and is concentrated in areas of the brain that are concerned with movement. A deficiency of dopamine can lead to Parkinson's disease. Too much dopamine is associated with schizophrenia. Other neurotransmitters include serotonin (5-hydroxytrypt-amine), adrenaline (also called epinephrine) and noradrenaline (norepinephrine). All of these neurotrans-mitters have effects in other parts of the body as well as in the brain. For example, adrenaline is produced by the adrenal glands just above the kidneys as well as at the ends of neurones in the brain. It causes the heart rate, blood pressure and blood sugar level to increase, preparing the body for 'fight or flight'. Adrenaline has a profound effect on mood, and thrill seekers crave it. Serotonin, too, has an important effect on our bodies as well as on our brains. It acts as a vasoconstrictor – a chemical that causes blood vessels to contract, reducing blood flow – but it also affects our mood and, indirectly, our perceptions. An excess of serotonin in the brain can produce nausea and migraines, for example. Having too little serotonin is one cause of depression. Post-mortem investigations of suicide victims and samples of the fluid from the spinal cords of depressed patients have revealed a deficit of serotonin, and the injection into a patient of a substance that breaks down serotonin can actually cause depression.

All the neurotransmitters mentioned are examples of a class of compounds called monoamines, and they have very similar molecular structures. In fact, the monoamines are related to each other in another way: adrenaline is made from noradrenaline, which is made from dopamine. Neurotransmitters are very important in the functioning of the brain, and in particular in making us feel good or not so good. Most illicit as well as medicinal drugs directly affect the production or inhibition of one or more neurotransmitters, or their uptake into the neurones either side of the synapses.

Where does MAO and thrill-seeking behaviour fit into this picture of synapses and neurotransmitters? MAO breaks down the monoamine neurotransmitters mentioned above. Specifically, it removes a part of the neurotransmitter molecules, rendering the molecules inactive. This is particularly important at synapses, where MAO 'mops up' after a nerve impulse has passed through. Both versions of MAO – A and B – are found in some of the cells that fill the spaces between neurones in the brain, the so-called glial (meaning 'glue') cells. From there, they can easily clean up the neurotransmitters released by nearby neurones. It seems that if the brain has too much MAO, the neurotransmitters do not work as effectively as they should, and this can lead to depression or lethargy. Since the late 1950s, drugs that inhibit MAO's activity have been used to treat people suffering from depression. The first 'MAO inhibitor' drug was called iproniazid. This drug was originally tested as a treatment for tuberculosis, but its use for that purpose was stopped when it was shown to produce euphoria in the patients who took it. In 1952, researchers found that iproniazid inhibited the action of MAO, and so they proposed that it could be used to treat depression. Its use began in 1958, but was halted after it was found to cause damage to the liver. However, since then, MAO inhibitors have become a major class of antidepressant drugs, and includes isocarboxazid (sold as Marplan). Most MAO inhibitors are generally used as a second line of attack because MAO inhibitors often have undesired side effects, and the exact mechanism by which they work is not very well understood. The first line of attack is normally to administer tricyclic antidepressants, which include imipramine (sold as Janimine and Tofranil). These work in a similar way to MAO inhibitors, by reducing the inactivation of certain neurotransmitters. The drug Prozac (fluoxetine) works in a different way again. It is one of a class of substances called SSRIs (selective serotonin re-uptake inhibitors), that prevents serotonin from being reabsorbed from the synapses, making them more active. Tranquillizers such as diazepam (Valium) work by enhancing the action of inhibitory neurotransmitters, such as gamma-aminobutyric acid. In this way, tranquillizers help to allow neurones to communicate more effectively.

Just as high concentrations of MAO have been associated with depression, many studies, including those carried out by Yu and Carrasco, have shown that low concentrations of the enzyme are associated with thrill-seeking behaviour. This behaviour crops up as a desire for novelty, stimulation or excitement, in many areas of life other than in dangerous sports. Carrasco himself has carried out other studies involving MAO. In 1994 he and his colleagues conducted a study of compulsive, or pathological, gamblers. He used several measurements of personality, including Zuckerman's Sensation Seeking Scale mentioned earlier, and took measurements of MAO B concentration in blood platelets from pathological gamblers and from members of a control group. As you might expect, the risk-taking, sensation-seeking gamblers had lower concentrations of MAO B in their blood than members of the control group.

Many other studies have highlighted a link between alcohol or drug abuse and low concentrations of MAO B, with care being taken to make sure that the drugs themselves had not affected the production of MAO B. In one study, blood taken from the umbilical cords joining newborn babies to their mothers was measured for MAO content. Babies with low MAO levels were found to be more physically active than those with normal levels. Studies have also been conducted in animals – monkeys and rats with low MAO B levels are more active and playful, and tend to sleep a good deal less. All in all, studies have shown, with varying degrees of certainty, that low concentrations of MAO B are associated with all of the following: sensation seeking, impulsiveness and 'monotony avoidance', job instability, poor academic performance, childhood hyperactivity, recreational drug use (particularly alcohol), defiance of punishment, extroversion, and a preference for highly varied sexual experiences.

The most likely explanation of MAO B's apparent importance in our behaviour involves the enzyme's ability to 'mop up' after neurotransmitters. If there is not enough MAO, the neurotransmitters hang around after they have been used, and can cause a kind of over-stimulation of neurones by allowing too many nerve signals to pass through. This may lead to hyperactivity in the brain, and this can pass on to a person's behaviour. Another possibility is that low levels of MAO are the effect and not the cause. The amount of MAO produced may be an indication of how much neurotransmitter is being produced. In this case, individuals who produce only a little neurotransmitter in a given situation will want to over-stimulate themselves, to give their brain a certain level of satisfaction.

T time

MAO is not the whole story in the quest to understand thrill seekers. Looking at the biochemistry of people whom personality tests highlight as 'type T' thrill seekers provides more clues in the quest to understand why the human brain takes risks. Many of these people have levels of the neurotransmitter dopamine that are higher than average. Dopamine is the 'feel good' neurotransmitter. In 1998 researchers at the University of California, Los Angeles, discovered an important link between thrill-seeking behaviour and dopamine receptors, which are vital in the transmission of nerve impulses across certain synapses in the brain. Dopamine receptors are like slots that dopamine molecules fit into on the receiving side of a synapse. In other words, dopamine molecules released by a nerve impulse that arrives at the first neurone burst across the synapse and attach to the second neurone, as described above. The dopamine receptors are very specific – only dopamine molecules can fit into them. When they do slot in, yet another chain of events occurs that results in tiny holes on the receiving neurone opening up, allowing positive ions to flow in. It is these ions that instigate the nerve impulse in the receiving neurone.

Until the early 1990s, three particular types of dopamine receptor had been identified. The fourth, named D4DR, was discovered in 1991, and a few years later it was found that there are several different versions of the gene responsible for manufacturing this receptor. So in 1995 a team of geneticists based at the Sara Herzog Hospital in Jerusalem and the Ben Gurion University in Beersheva set about investigating this gene. They wanted to find out whether people's personalities might be in part determined by which version of the D4DR gene they possess. In particular, did having one version of this gene make people more sensation seeking?

They selected at random 124 people, and subjected them to personality tests as well as genetic tests to determine which version of the D4DR gene they possessed. They found that people with one version of the gene scored 10 per cent higher in their sensation-seeking scores than those who had the other version. This result has been repeated in several studies in several countries, including the one in Los Angeles, and this genetic basis for at least part of sensation-seeking behaviour is well established. It has been discovered that people with one version of the gene have only half the density of the dopamine receptors in their synapses as people with the other. The team in Los Angeles looked at two different dopamine receptor genes, D2DR and D4DR. They carried out genetic and psychological tests on 119 boys aged twelve years, and found that boys who had a particular version of each of the two genes had significantly higher sensation-seeking scores than the other boys. In addition, they found that boys who had only one of the versions in question had slightly higher sensation-seeking scores than the average, but slightly lower than the boys with the relevant versions of both the genes.

The connection between sensation seeking and dopamine is clear. But so is the link between sensation seeking and addictive behaviour such as alcoholism and drug abuse. Further evidence of this second link comes from experiments on rats at the US National Institute of Drug Abuse (NIDA). In 1995, researchers funded by NIDA and working at the University of Kentucky found that the same 'reward pathways' in the rats' brains were involved in the search for novel experiences as are involved in drug-taking. In the first of two experiments, they found that rats' desire for novelty could be dampened down by administering a drug that affected the action of dopamine receptors in the reward pathways, the main one of which is in the limbic system of the brain. In the second, they showed that when rats were engaged in novel activities, such as investigating previously unexplored chambers in a maze, the same reward pathways were stimulated.

The limbic system is involved in many brain functions, including emotion in humans. It includes brain structures such as the hippocampus and the amygdalae. The fact that the major reward pathways, sometimes referred to as the reward cascade, are located in the limbic system was discovered in the 1950s, by American psychologists James Olds and Peter Milner. In their experiments, Olds and Milner connected the limbic systems of living rats to a low-power source of electricity. The rats could stimulate the electrodes, to deliver a burst of electricity to the limbic system, by pressing a lever. The researchers found that the rats pressed the levers repeatedly and continuously, up to five thousand times every hour. They also found that being allowed to press the lever would be a more than adequate reward to encourage rats to solve problems like finding their way around mazes. Later, Olds went on to perform similar experiments in human subjects, who reported pleasurable, even orgasmic feelings when regions of their limbic systems were stimulated. They felt light-headed and their minds were cleared of any negative thoughts they had prior to stimulation. Alcohol, nicotine and cocaine are known to promote the release of dopamine (and another neurotransmitter called acetylcholine) in the reward pathways of the brain, and this explains why they can become addictive: they excite the reward pathways, and reduce the craving for reward in the human brain. Unfortunately for smokers, cocaine users and alcoholics, the brain 'habituates' to the effects of these substances and, after prolonged use, more and more of these substances is required to produce the same effect.

The convincing evidence that increased dopamine activity and reduced levels of MAO are important factors in thrill-seeking behaviours and in drug addiction or dependency could be worrying. It does not mean that all people who engage in extreme sports are at risk of becoming drug addicts. However, it may well be that extreme sports can be a replacement for drug dependency – perhaps the same urge for thrills can be satisfied in either activity. Could BASE jumping and other extreme sports be an effective way of avoiding drug dependency?

In 1995 the National Institute of Drug Addiction created a novel media campaign that was aimed at young sensation seekers. The campaign was based around a booklet and television adverts. One of the scientists involved in the campaign, Dr Lewis Donohow of the University of Kentucky, said that, because sensation seekers have different perceptions of risk, 'ads using scare tactics may actually enhance the attractiveness of drug use for high sensation seekers'. Particularly worrying for children of alcoholics or drug addicts is the fact that a tendency for alcohol or other drug dependency is at least partly inherited. This may lead some alcoholics to blame their inheritance – 'my genes made me do it' – but that is little comfort in the face of some of the social implications of addiction.

Some studies have shown that intervention in the reward pathways in the brain can be effective in helping alcoholics to stop drinking. When a compound called bromocryptine was administered to alcoholics, it was found in many cases to reduce the craving and make it easier for the alcoholics to kick their habit. Bromocryptine is a dopamine agonist, which means that it can stimulate the same pathways as dopamine itself. According to a report by behavioural geneticist Kenneth Blum and his colleagues, there are about 18 million alcoholics in the USA, 28 million children of alcoholics, 25 million people who are addicted to nicotine and about 6 million cocaine addicts. The report suggests that all these behaviours, and various behavioural disorders such as attention deficit disorder (ADD or ADHD), and perhaps thrill seeking, can all be thought of as one condition: 'reward deficiency syndrome'.

Blum and his colleagues foresee effective prevention and treatment of alcoholism and other 'reward deficiencies', as well as an understanding that these behaviours are not entirely the fault of the individual. This, they say, will remove the social stigma of such conditions. However, this sort of idea could be used to restrict people's freedom. In the future it may be possible to screen babies – or even embryos – for the 'genes for alcoholism'. Alternatively, these genes could even be genetically engineered out of the genome. There is no serious suggestion of doing this, and indeed some of the same biochemistry that can lead to addiction can also lead to thrill-seeking behaviour. And thrill-seeking behaviour is important: the world needs people who are full of energy, who are creative and dynamic. These are the sorts of traits that we find in thrill seekers and risk takers. People who engage in extreme sports have often been labelled as 'having a death wish'. Quoted in the magazine *US News*, Marvin Zuckerman says that this cannot be true: 'If these people were real death wishers, they wouldn't bother with safety precautions. The death wish is a myth made up by those who aren't high-sensation seekers who can't understand the rewards.'

There do seem to be biological causes of sensation-seeking behaviour, involving neurotransmitters such as dopamine and adrenaline, and the enzyme MAO. For people who are predisposed by their genes and their biochemistry to be sensation seekers, the world has become worryingly safe. BASE jumper Elliot certainly thinks so: 'Imagine jumping off a housing tower block ... your toes are two inches over the edge of the roof ... you push out, arch your back, and all of a sudden you start accelerating down the side of this building. You see the lights start to speed up as you fall. All of a sudden – crack – the canopy opens. Once you've landed, you look up at this building and there might be three or four hundred people living there ... content to sit watching television ... I wouldn't want to live if that was me.'

THIN AIR
... in search of oxygen...

Climbing Mount Everest is one of the ultimate human challenges. The mountain's peak sits more than eight kilometres (5.5 miles) above sea level, well above most of the cloud tops. It is cold and remote, and the climb is hard and dangerous. The hardships and the dangers are intensified by the effects of a decrease in oxygen in climbers' blood. On top of Mount Everest, a climber takes in about one-third as much oxygen with each breath as at sea level. Oxygen is needed by all of the tissues of our body, but the organ that uses the most is the brain. What happens to the brain when it receives less oxygen than it needs? In 1997 a team of climbers, led by mountaineer and film maker David Breashears, conducted a special expedition to explore and document the effects of breathing 'thin air'. The expedition was sponsored by the public television science series *NOVA*, produced in the United States by the WGBH Science Unit.

On top of the world
David Breashears had already three times reached the summit of Mount Everest before embarking on this scientific mission. In one of those ascents, in 1996, he made a remarkable film of the mountain using an IMAX camera – which produces a huge, high quality, wide-angle picture – so that others might share some of the experience of being on top of the world. At the same time that Breashears was

making his IMAX film, eight climbers died in a single day. The tragedy was caused partly by blizzard conditions, but also partly by the number of people who were on the mountain. Sometimes bottlenecks form at certain parts of the main route up to the summit, due to the large numbers of climbers. In 1993 a total of 129 people made it to the top of Mount Everest – a record that is likely to be broken in the next few years. There is ample evidence of the increasing numbers of visitors to this hostile place: as well as Base Camp, there are discarded or abandoned tent poles, tent pegs and oxygen bottles at some of the four camps where climbers stop for a night or two en route to the summit. And, scattered at various points along the route, there are human remains – when climbers die on the mountain, it is usually not practical to recover the bodies and carry them down for a proper burial.

For every six successful summits of Mount Everest, one person dies. Reduced oxygen supply to the brain can cause confusion and loss of co-ordination. The tragedy that killed eight people in 1996 – along with many of the other deaths on Mount Everest – was probably also due to the effects on the brain of breathing the tenuous atmosphere at high altitude. This made Breashears's expedition and experiment all the more important.

Joining David Breashears on this scientific voyage were Ed Viesturs and David Carter. Viesturs is one of the most experienced mountaineers in the world – before joining this expedition, he had already climbed Mount Everest four times, three of them without supplemental oxygen. David Carter was returning to the mountain after an unsuccessful attempt to climb to the summit six years earlier. Another key member of the team was Jangbu Sherpa, who did not take part in the scientific experiments but headed the team of Sherpas supporting the effort. Jangbu had climbed Mount Everest twice before, including in 1996 when he assisted Breashears's film-making expedition. Also part of the team was Pete Athans, who was to operate a digital video camera and also take tests. At the time of writing, Athans is the only non-Sherpa to reach the peak of Mount Everest six times. Also part of the expedition was Dr Howard Donner, the expedition doctor, who was to remain at Base Camp, 3,490 metres (11,400 feet) below the summit.

At a staggering 8,850 metres, the higher of Mount Everest's two peaks is the highest solid ground above sea level on which you can stand anywhere in the world. When asked what the height of Mount Everest is, many people will quote a different value: 29,028 feet (actually 8,848 metres). This figure is familiar because climbers tend to give values of height in feet, and so the figure of '29,028 feet' has stuck in people's minds since it was announced in 1954 by the Indian Bureau of Measurement. However, those people will now have to learn a new figure: in November 1999 the measurement of 29,035 feet (8,850 metres) was officially recognized by the American National Geographic Society. The new, highly accurate measurement was taken in May 1999, by an American team led by Pete Athans using high-tech GPS (Global Positioning System) satellite navigation equipment. A recent geological study has shown that Everest is increasing by as much as three centimetres per year, due to the same forces that have been forming the mountain for the past sixty million years.

The 'new' height of Mount Everest is not the only thing that may come as a surprise. Although the mountain is the highest point on the Earth above sea level, it is not the furthest from the centre of the Earth. This is because our planet is not perfectly round – it is an oblate spheroid, a slightly flattened sphere. Its diameter at the equator is 42 kilometres (26 miles) greater than its diameter from pole to pole. So the peak of a mountain in Ecuador, Chimborazo, which sits only one degree south of the equator, is actually further from the centre of the Earth, although it is more than eight thousand feet (2,440 metres) shorter than Mount

Everest as measured from sea level. And, perhaps even more surprisingly, Mount Everest is not even the tallest landform as measured from its base to its peak. That honour goes to a huge, snow-capped volcano, Mauna Kea, that rises out of the ocean in Hawaii. If you could move it on to dry land and take it to Nepal, Mauna Kea would stand nearly three thousand feet (900 metres) taller than Mount Everest.

Despite these peculiarities about the height of Mount Everest – known as Chomolungma ('goddess mother of the world') in Tibet and Sagarmatha ('goddess of the sky') in Nepal – it remains the aim of many climbers to conquer this mountain. With its peak well within the 'death zone', above about eight thousand metres (26,000 feet), in which climbers become out of breath just breathing, it makes a perfect natural laboratory in which to study the effects of oxygen deprivation on the brain. The brain constitutes only 2.5 per cent of the body's mass, but uses up 20 per cent of the energy. The source of this energy is the process of aerobic respiration, which involves the reaction of glucose (a type of sugar) in the blood with oxygen.

It's a gas
Oxygen – denoted by the chemical symbol 'O' – is the most abundant element in the Earth's crust. This is because it occurs, combined with other elements, in the rocks that make up the crust, such as limestone (calcium carbonate, $CaCO_3$) and quartz (silicon dioxide, SiO_2). It is also the most abundant element (by weight) in the oceans, lakes and rivers: every drop of water is made of countless oxygen and hydrogen atoms joined together in groups of three called water molecules (H_2O). When pure, it is a gas at room temperature – the oxygen atoms join in pairs to form oxygen molecules (O_2). Oxygen becomes a liquid if cooled to below minus 183 degrees C (minus 297 degrees F). The resulting liquid is pale blue. Cool it still further, to minus 218 degrees C (minus 361 F), and it becomes a bright red solid.

Oxygen was discovered in the 1770s, at a time when several eminent scientists, mostly in Europe, were experimenting with the physical and chemical characteristics of gases. In 1772 the Swedish chemist Karl Scheele produced oxygen gas by heating other substances. And in England two years later, Joseph Priestley discovered oxygen in the same way – he noted that a candle would burn remarkably well in the gas. An existing scientific theory postulated that when matter burns it releases a hypothetical substance called phlogiston. Priestley assumed that the reason the candle burned so well in the newly discovered gas was that it had a great affinity for phlogiston. And he guessed that this might be because the gas had no phlogiston, so he named it 'dephlogisticated air'. It was a French chemist, Antoine-Laurent Lavoisier, who realized the role of this gas in burning and in respiration. When a substance burns, the atoms and molecules of which it is made combine with oxygen – this is the real reason that Priestley's candles burned so well in the pure but as yet unnamed gas.

Scientists before Lavoisier had noticed that most substances lose weight as they burn – candles, for example, grow smaller as they burn. They assumed that the reduction in weight was associated with the release of phlogiston. However, some substances – in particular, metals – actually gain weight when they burn, and this posed a problem for the phlogiston theory. Lavoisier was the first person to realize the importance of oxygen in the burning process, and that in some cases – such as a candle – the products of burning were released into the atmosphere, therefore explaining the loss of weight. In other cases, the oxygen remained, chemically combined with the substance, and this explained the increase in weight. If you burn iron wool, for example, the resulting compound, called iron oxide, is heavier than the original iron wool, due to the oxygen that has combined with the iron. In one stroke, then, Lavoisier had overturned the phlogiston theory, and oxygen had been recognized as a very important element. He realized, too, that water was the product of hydrogen gas burning.

He extended his studies of oxygen to bodily processes: he observed, for example, that birds kept in sealed, oxygen-filled cases lived longer than birds in atmospheric air, which contains less oxygen. Unknown to Lavoisier, the oxygen that the birds inhaled was used in the tissues of the birds' bodies, to release energy, in the process of respiration. In fact, respiration and burning have a lot in common. A burning candle releases heat and light energy, as oxygen (O) from the air combines with the atoms of carbon (C) and hydrogen (H) of which the candle is made, to produce carbon dioxide (CO_2) and water (H_2O). In a similar way, oxygen carried by the blood combines with glucose ($C_6H_{12}O_6$) in a kind of burning reaction, releasing energy for use by the muscles and the brain, and producing water and carbon dioxide as waste products.

The oxygen required for respiration comes from the atmosphere, a little of which you take in every time you inhale. The atmosphere is made up of a mixture of many different types of molecules, all dashing around at high speed, bouncing off each other and anything else that gets in their way. Where air molecules bombard a surface, they exert pressure – a balloon stays inflated because the air inside it is at higher pressure than the air outside it, for example. This is because the collisions of billions of air molecules against the inside of the rubber produce greater force than the collisions of molecules on the outside. And although you cannot feel it, the air at sea level presses against you with a force about equal to the weight of a kilogram bag of sugar on each square centimetre. When you breathe in, your chest expands, reducing the pressure of the air inside your lungs; higher pressure air from outside rushes in. The density of the atmosphere – a measure of the mass of air present in a particular volume – decreases with altitude, too. At sea level, one cubic metre of air has a mass of 1.22 kilograms. At the summit of Mount Everest, the density of the air is less than half a kilogram per cubic metre. The reason for this difference in mass is that the air molecules are more spread out at high altitudes. Air at sea level – at the bottom of the atmosphere – is 'squashed' by the weight of air above it. In each cubic centimetre of air molecules at sea level, there are about twenty-five million million million air molecules. At the top of Mount Everest, however, there are 'only' about nine million million million air molecules in each cubic centimetre. About twenty-one per cent of them are oxygen molecules – this is true at any altitude. You take in about three litres (3,000 cubic centimetres) of air with each breath. So, at the summit of Mount Everest, about five thousand million million million oxygen molecules rush into your lungs each time you inhale.

What happens to oxygen molecules once they are inside your lungs? Most of them are expelled again when you exhale, but some of them make it into the alveoli, tiny spaces in your lungs. If you imagine a lung as an upside-down tree, the alveoli are the leaves. And just as leaves are involved in exchanging gases between a tree and the surrounding air, gas exchange takes place in the alveoli. Molecules of oxygen pass from the air through the very thin membrane of each alveolus, and into the blood. Some of the molecules dissolve directly into the blood plasma, but most of them attach to molecules of haemoglobin, a pigment found in red blood cells. Haemoglobin is blue when it carries no oxygen but becomes red as soon as oxygen molecules – four per haemoglobin molecule – are attached. In fact, red blood cells are red only when they are carrying oxygen. At the same time that oxygen is passing into your blood, carbon dioxide – one of the waste products of the reaction of sugars with oxygen – passes from the blood to the air in the alveoli, and out into the atmosphere when you breathe out. The blood, with a fresh supply of oxygen and having rid itself of much of the carbon dioxide, then passes from the lungs to the heart, from where it is pumped around the body. Very little oxygen is actually stored in the body, so if breathing stops, or there is no oxygen in the air, the result is death within a few minutes.

The importance of oxygen in the brain is highlighted by modern medical scanning techniques called functional MRI (magnetic resonance imaging) and PET (positron emission tomography). In one form of PET, a special glucose solution is injected into a patient. Glucose reacts with blood oxygen to release energy required by living cells. The molecules of glucose in the injected solution are radioactive, and decay by releasing particles called positrons. When these particles collide with electrons in the patient's brain, they release gamma radiation (electromagnetic radiation like X-rays), which is detected by sensors positioned around the body. Computer analysis of what the detectors pick up show where glucose is most concentrated, and so which tissues are demanding the most energy, using the most oxygen. PET brain scans can help to identify which areas of the brain are most involved in certain mental tasks. Functional MRI can also visualize which areas of the brain are demanding the most oxygen: it discriminates between haemoglobin molecules with oxygen and those without. The images created by an MRI scanner show areas with high oxygen content, and therefore where oxygen demands are highest. MRI and PET have begun to unravel the mysteries of what part of the brain does what during different kinds of task.

In short supply

As we have seen, each breath at high altitude takes in less oxygen, at a lower pressure, than each breath at sea level. The first effect of breathing air at altitude is that less oxygen reaches the haemoglobin in the blood. The tissues of the body – including those in the brain – are then supplied with less oxygen than they require, a condition known as hypoxia. The lower pressure of air at altitude means that the air presses less hard against the membranes of the alveoli – this is why less oxygen is absorbed into the blood. High-altitude climbers are well aware of some of the milder physiological effects of hypoxia, which together are known as mountain sickness, or altitude sickness. As mountaineers stay at high altitudes for relatively short periods of time, symptoms are normally short-lived. For that reason, mountain sickness is normally referred to as acute rather than chronic. The symptoms of acute mountain sickness include dizziness, severe headaches, lack of appetite, impaired judgement and even hallucinations. When crossing the dangerous crevasses and climbing up the hazardous icefalls of the world's highest mountains, these symptoms can put climbers at great risk. Many of the deaths of high-altitude climbers are a direct result of the loss of judgement associated with hypoxia; the main rationale behind the study carried out by Breashears and his colleagues was to understand the effects of hypoxia on the brain.

This is not the only study to have investigated these effects. Several others have measured various aspects of cognitive performance in experiments carried out at high altitude, while others have investigated the effects of hypoxia in sea-level experiments. It is possible to induce hypoxia at sea level by supplying someone with air at a lower pressure or air that is deficient in oxygen. Some such studies are carried out to assess the physiological and psychological effects of hypoxia on people who commute to high-altitude areas – most astronomers, for example, work in telescopes situated well above the light-obscuring pollution of cities, high up on mountains, and miners in several locations in South America who live near sea level but work in mines at locations as high as 4,500 metres (14,800 feet). Other studies are conducted with air or space travel in mind – many aeroplanes cruise at altitudes greater than the height of Mount Everest. Of course, aeroplanes are pressurized containers, so pilots and passengers do not breathe air from the atmosphere at that height. However, the air inside the cabin of an aeroplane is not pressurized to simulate the atmosphere at sea level. It is not uncommon for the air inside cabins to be at the same pressure as the atmosphere at an altitude of 2,440 metres (8,000 feet). Most people do not have symptoms of altitude sickness or loss of cognitive function at this height – these signs usually appear higher than about three thousand metres (10,000 feet).

It has been shown that mountain sickness and mental dysfunction due to hypoxia affect different people in different ways, so some people might feel slight effects of hypoxia during an aeroplane flight. If those people were pilots – who rely on quick reactions and clarity of mind – then safety could be compromised, so this kind of research is important. Other research – including that carried out by Breashears and his team – is aimed at examining the effects of hypoxia on mountaineers, basically to understand the relationship between mental dysfunction and climbing tragedies. This is not true of all such studies: in 1993, Philip Lieberman, Professor of Cognitive and Linguistic Science at Brown University, Rhode Island, conducted a study of climbers on Mount Everest to test his theory about the evolution of speech. From the fact that the mental dysfunction of climbers at altitude covers a range of abilities, he concluded that speech involves archaic brain mechanisms, involved with muscle control, as well as mechanisms more recent in evolutionary history, such as the elements of language. In his book *Eve Spoke: Human Language and Human Evolution* Lieberman says that the results of the cognitive tests taken by the climbers at altitude 'suggest a linkage between the neural mechanisms implicated in speech motor control and syntax'. There is more to studying the effects of the air we breathe than you might have thought.

It is only in recent years – with a sophisticated understanding of the processes of respiration – that we have been able to study the effects of hypoxia in a scientific way. But humans have been aware of the effects of breathing at high altitude for at least two thousand years. In about AD20 a Chinese general described the routes taken by travellers in the Karakoram mountain range in China, in which is found the popular peak K2. According to the account, the routes were named according to how they made the travellers feel – there was Mount Greater Headache and Fever Hill, for example. The general's report described how people and some animals experienced feverish symptoms when they were climbing over the higher parts of some of these routes. When hot-air ballooning became popular at the end of the eighteenth century, more people began to fly to increasingly higher altitudes. Balloonists' reports of the strange effects of breathing rarefied (low-density) air were sometimes conflicting. Many balloonists reported suffering from headaches and vomiting – the symptoms of acute mountain sickness – but some actually thought they might gain some benefit from breathing rarefied air. One even went as far as to suggest taking chronically sick people up in balloons to high altitudes, as a form of medical treatment. The idea that the fresh air at high altitudes can have a therapeutic effect persists today: for 5,000 US dollars you can buy the 'Altitude Tent', and benefit from increased production of red blood cells and improved lung performance. And indeed, there is an increase in the production of oxygen-carrying red blood cells and an increase in lung performance when a person breathes in less oxygen than they need. The price tag may seem a little steep, but the manufacturers' claim that it can save mountaineers time and money by allowing them to acclimatize before they arrive at Base Camp.

The first person to investigate scientifically the link between the symptoms of acute mountain sickness and oxygen deprivation was German explorer Alexander von Humboldt. In the first few years of the nineteenth century he climbed several high mountains in South America. His assault on Chimborazo in Ecuador, which fell about three hundred metres (1,000 feet) short of the summit, was a high-altitude climbing record for nearly thirty years. All Humboldt's climbs were achieved without oxygen supplies – pure, bottled oxygen was not available until the early 1900s – and Humboldt described the symptoms now diagnosed as acute mountain sickness. It was not until 1937 that the medical community recognized the condition.

The physiological effects of acute mountain sickness – headaches, nausea and fatigue – are no doubt related to the increase in breathing, blood pressure and heart rate and the change in the levels of various enzymes and hormones that are instigated in climbers when their bodies receive less oxygen than normal. The effects of oxygen deprivation on the brain vary from mild mental dysfunction, through permanent damage, to death. Most human cells can survive without a constant supply of oxygen. For example, muscle cells in a sprinter's legs derive energy temporarily using a reaction that does not involve oxygen. In fact, whenever any muscle cell is working it is always deriving its energy without involving oxygen – the oxygen becomes involved after the muscle stops working. Brain cells cannot release energy this way, and die quickly in the absence of oxygen. Permanent brain damage can result from lack of oxygen at birth for just a few minutes, for example. Strokes are caused largely by a lack of oxygen to the brain. A stroke causes massive damage to the brain by interrupting the blood supply there – because a blood clot blocks an artery, for instance. The symptoms exhibited by stroke victims can include lack of co-ordination or even paralysis of an area of the body (or the mind) associated with the part of the brain that is damaged. The lack of oxygen due to the interruption of blood supply is a major cause of these symptoms, as large numbers of neurones may die. While a near-total loss of oxygen supply to the brain can result in permanent or semi-permanent brain damage, what might be the effects of the slight reduction in supply experienced by climbers at altitude? If oxygen supply to the whole brain is reduced, you would expect a general reduction in a person's mental faculties. This would perhaps manifest itself as a general, but temporary, loss of co-ordination, memory, comprehension and language capability – all of which are very important to mountaineers at high altitudes. Measuring and cataloguing these effects will improve safety for climbers – that is the aim of studies such as the one carried out by Breashears and his team.

While breathing less oxygen than you need is harmful, breathing pure oxygen or air at high pressure often has therapeutic effects. Oxygen tents are transportable cabinets in which oxygen-enriched air circulates. Patients suffering from respiratory complaints or heart disease may spend time in these cabinets, which are also controlled for temperature and humidity. Between 30 and 50 per cent of the air inside the tent is oxygen gas – much greater than in atmospheric air. An incubator is very similar, and is used to house babies born prematurely so that they have a greater chance of surviving and avoiding brain damage or other disorders. And another similar idea is the hyperbaric chamber – a large tank filled with air at a pressure higher than in the atmosphere at sea level. The oxygen molecules that rush into the lungs when you breathe such air are pushed through the membranes in the lungs' alveoli more forcefully than in normal air. There are many uses of hyperbaric chambers, including treatment for decompression illness. This dangerous condition occurs when a person who has been in a high-pressure environment – such as deep under the ocean – moves too quickly to a lower-pressure environment. What happens under high pressure is that gases are forced to dissolve into the blood and then into the body's tissues. Moving to lower pressure slowly allows these gases to pass back into the blood and then out into the lungs, causing no problems. If decompression is too quick, however, the gases do not have time to pass into the blood, and instead they form dangerous bubbles in the tissues. The most problematic gas is nitrogen, since it constitutes more than seventy-five per cent of the atmosphere and is not used up by the body's tissues, as oxygen is when it reacts with glucose to produce energy. When a deep-sea diver comes to the surface too quickly, enough nitrogen forms tiny bubbles in various tissues to cause major problems. A diver with decompression illness is often described as having 'the bends', because the bubbles of nitrogen under the skin can cause swelling that means that joints cannot be bent or unbent. Bubbles that form in the brain or the spinal cord can cause serious disorientation and paralysis or loss of co-ordination.

Hyperbaric chambers can also help babies born with heart defects. Such babies can be placed in hyperbaric chambers before an operation, which may give them a better chance of survival and recovery. Hyperbaric chambers that contain pure high-pressure oxygen also have an additional range of uses. Some harmful bacteria, inside or on the surface of the body, cannot live in high concentrations of oxygen, for example, and oxygen is sometimes used as a fast healer. Breathing inside such a chamber, you take in more oxygen than normal, and at higher pressure. The result is that the concentration of oxygen dissolved in the blood plasma rises dramatically – by as much as two thousand per cent. This does not mean that the total amount of oxygen in the blood increases by that amount – most of the oxygen carried by the blood is attached to haemoglobin molecules in the red blood cells. One cannot force more than four molecules of oxygen on to each haemoglobin molecule, and increasing the atmospheric pressure will do nothing to increase the numbers of red blood cells. However, the extra oxygen dissolved in the plasma will be delivered to the various tissues of the body – what might be the benefits of this? Some people use hyperbaric oxygen chambers to treat stroke, coma and traumatic brain injuries. The idea is that the extra oxygen encourages the regeneration of neurones in the damaged brain – though not everyone believes that this approach actually works. Another controversial application of hyperbaric oxygen tanks is to help people lose weight. Here, the idea is that increased oxygen in the blood will increase metabolic rate, to 'burn calories'. Other examples are 'smart pills' and 'smart drinks'. Their manufacturers claim that they enhance mental performance because they contain large amounts of oxygen, or increase oxygen delivery to brain cells. And there are increasingly popular 'oxygen bars', where people socialize and pay to inhale pure oxygen.

Testing time
So much for high-pressure, high-density air, oxygen bars and smart pills. In order to investigate how the effects of too little oxygen relate to altitude and to oxygen concentration in climbers' blood, Breashears and his team were to conduct a number of physiological and mental tests. They would carry out these tests at sea level, at several different eleva- tions on their way up to the summit of Mount Everest, and – if they made it to the top – at the summit itself. The tests at sea level were baseline tests: the results of these would be used as points of reference against which to compare the results of the tests taken at altitude. The baseline tests were carried out at the University of Washington Harbourview Medical Centre in Seattle. There, Dr Brownie Schoene first subjected Breashears, Viesturs and Carter to MRI brain scans, which also allowed the doctor to anticipate some of the effects that being at high altitudes might have on the climbers' brains. First, Schoene carried out a scan on each member of the climbing team while they were resting – sim- ply lying still on the table, inside the scanner's strong magnetic field. Next, he scanned them again while the climbers were over-breathing – hyperventilating. Each climber

had to lie down in the brain scanner and purposely hyper-ventilate for twenty minutes. Breathing at altitude would be laboured and rapid like this, so this second set of scans would show what chemical changes might take place in the brain at altitude. The scans also enabled Schoene to measure the volumes of the climbers' brains – there is some evidence that repeated exposure to high-altitude can actually reduce the size of the brain slightly. Another set of MRI scans would be carried out after the expedition, allowing Schoene and physiologist Peter Hackett to check whether the climbers' brains did shrink as a result of their high-altitude experiences.

After the MRI scans, the climbers underwent other physiological tests, including spirometry – measurement of lung capacity – and measurement of HVR (hypoxic ventilatory response), which is a gauge of how well and how quickly the body adjusts to breathing in less oxygen than normal. The climbers' HVRs were measured by testing the blood for 'oxygen saturation' and by monitoring the heart rate and breathing rate. At sea level, your blood is normally totally saturated with oxygen, meaning that the haemoglobin molecules in your red blood cells are carrying as much oxygen as they can. The oxygen saturation is measured as a percentage and depends upon the concentration of oxygen in the plasma of the blood. The higher the concentration of oxygen in the plasma, the more oxygen is taken up by the haemoglobin in the red blood cells. As you would expect, oxygen saturation falls as people breathe at altitude; this is because the lower atmospheric pressure there means that less oxygen dissolves in the plasma. During the tests for HVR, each climber was made to breathe through a mouthpiece – the air supply was gradually changed to simulate the air they would breathe at high altitude. The climbers' oxygen saturation levels dropped to around seventy per cent, and heart rate rose from around sixty-five to over 100. This is a normal response to breathing air with lower-than-normal pressure and density. Each climber was also tested to gauge the maximum amount of oxygen his body used when working flat out. On a treadmill, the climbers breathed through a mouthpiece that supplied them with normal sea-level air and measured the amount of oxygen their bodies demanded. All the climbers were found to be in excellent condition, ready for the physical challenges that awaited them on the mountain.

Psychometric tests were also conducted at the university, and would be repeated at altitude. These tests would not be able to come to any truly scientific conclusions about what hypoxia can do to the brain: the effects of general fatigue, lack of sleep, diet and climate, for example, would also probably affect the test results. However, the test results would add valuable data to existing findings about the effects of high altitudes on cognitive function. Psychometrics expert Gail Rosenbaum collected together standard tests that would give an indication of how clearly and quickly the climbers were thinking. During the baseline test session, she commented, 'What we will expect to see is that there is a slowing of speech; there'll be a slowing in reaction time; we may see a lot of mis-speaks; they won't say things quite the way they would at sea level; there'll be a lot of slurring and hesitation.'

There were five different types of test, each measuring a slightly different aspect of cognitive function. One test measured the climbers' attention: the climbers were asked to listen to a series of high and low tones, and state how many low tones were present in each case, ignoring the high tones. Another well-known psychometric test, called the Stroop test, measured flexibility in the climbers' thinking by investigating the ability to inhibit one of two responses. In the Stroop test, the person being tested looks at words printed in different colours, and has to say out loud the colour of the ink in each case. Each word is actually the name of a colour, but one that is different from the colour in which the word is printed – so, for example, the person might read the word 'RED' printed in green ink, and be asked what colour the ink is. The person's brain becomes conscious of two conflicting items – the colour of the ink and the word itself – but would be asked to state just one. Success in this task requires the person to choose the desired item and discard the other. 'That'll be fun at altitude,' David Carter joked as he took the Stroop test.

Some PET brain studies have shown that an area of the brain between the two cerebral hemispheres, called the anterior cingulate, demands energy during the Stroop test. If this region does not receive the oxygen it requires when this test is being taken, at high altitudes, perhaps test performance will be impaired. The third type of test comprised sets of simple true-or-false questions. This would provide a way of measuring mental speed. Statements such as 'Roast beef can be eaten' and 'Squirrels are usually sold in pairs' were included – they are very simple, so the time taken to give the answer is then a measure of mental speed, not of the level of cognitive ability. Rosenbaum expected that the climbers would take longer to answer at altitude. The fourth type of test – simple verbal puzzles – was also used to measure mental speed, but also to test verbal reasoning ability. Each puzzle took the form of a statement followed by a question – for example 'Charles beats David in a sprint; which man is faster?' The final type of test administered both at baseline and on the mountain was based on short-term memory and attention. The climbers were asked to listen to and then repeat sentences, such as 'Mike walked around the block three times until he had the nerve to knock on Carol's door'. Helping to conduct the physiological and psychological baseline tests was Dr Howard Donner, who would be going to Nepal with the climbers, as the expedition physician. From Base Camp, he was to keep in regular contact with the climbers, to record their blood saturation levels and heart rates and to conduct the psychometric tests.

To Base Camp

Early in April 1997 the team set off for the Himalayan mountains. The medical and scientific team was to stay at Base Camp, at an altitude of 5,360 metres (17,600 feet). In the early expeditions to climb Mount Everest, climbers had to trek for weeks just to reach Base Camp before they started their assault proper on the mountain. Nowadays, climbers are generally flown by helicopter from Kathmandu to Lukla, at an elevation of 2,440 metres (8,000 feet). The journey from there to Base Camp takes about ten days. Mount Everest is shaped somewhat like a pyramid, with three distinct faces – the north face, the east face and the south-west face. Most Everest expeditions approach the summit via the south-east ridge. There are three ridges that lead to the north face: the north-east ridge, the west ridge and the south-east ridge. David Breashears and his team elected to use the south-east ridge, which is the one most often used because it is the least precarious. Having said that, the ridge is still extremely dangerous, as it falls away sharply 3,000 metres (10,000 feet) on either side. Many climbers have died at this point of the climb. The danger is exacerbated, of course, by the effects of acute mountain sickness – the ridge is only 100 metres (330 feet) below the summit.

On the way up to the south-east ridge climbers generally stop at four camps, usually spending a few nights at each. This is so that they can acclimatize to the increase in altitude on moving from one camp to the next. The journey from Base Camp to Camp I – up through a treacherous icefall – is the most dangerous part of the climb. Camp I is situated on the gradual slope of a long glacier called the Western Cwm. From Camp I Sherpas ferry supplies to the higher camps. Camp II, at the top of the Western Cwm, is perhaps the most important of the camps. From here, climbers ascend one of the faces of a mountain called Lhotse – Mount Everest's next-door neighbour – before crossing the south-east ridge. Camps III and IV are situated at either side of the Lhotse Face. Camp IV – called the South Col – lies at the foot of the south-east ridge, and it is from there that climbers mount their final assault on the summit.

The route taken by most climbers up the mountain today – including Breashears and his team – is the same as that taken by the first people to make it to the summit, New Zealand climber Edmund Hillary and Sherpa Tenzing Norgay. Their historic journey was completed in May 1953, but several expeditions during the 1920s came very close to reaching the summit. Perhaps the most famous of these was the 1924 expedition in which the celebrated British climber George Mallory and his colleague Sandy Irvine tragically lost their lives. Mallory's body was discovered in May 1999 by a team of climbers, on a special recovery mission. The body was found jutting out of the snow below the north-east ridge, just 600 metres (2,000 feet) short of the summit. During that fateful mission, eight climbing assistants, mainly Sherpas, died during an avalanche.

Despite the obvious risks to which they put themselves, Sherpas have been an important part of every expedition on Mount Everest. The Sherpa people live both in Nepal and India, and number about a hundred and twenty thousand in total. About three thousand of these live in the Khumbu Valley in Nepal, which forms much of the approach route to Everest Base Camp. The Sherpa traditionally used yaks to carry goods such as wool for trade, and yaks are used to help carry much of the huge consignment of supplies required by Mount Everest expeditions from Lukla to Base Camp. The tented village that is Base Camp typically houses between three and four hundred people, comprising climbing parties, their guides and Sherpa support teams. Breashears and his team had a tent dedicated to the radio and scientific equipment they needed to record the results of the physiological and psychometric tests that the climbers would be undertaking.

Even at Base Camp, the dramatic physiological effects of being at high altitude could be felt. The expedition climbers – and the medical and scientific team – all experienced headaches and fatigue, and their blood oxygen saturation level was much lower than at sea level, at about seventy-five per cent. Oxygen saturations were measured using a hand-held device called a pulse oxymeter, which fits over a finger and gives an instant reading. It works by shining red and infrared light through the finger and detecting what proportion of each passes through. If only red light were used, then the device would indicate only the amount of oxygen-carrying haemoglobin present. By comparing the amounts of red and infrared light that pass through the finger, a pulse oxymeter is able to calculate the ratio of oxygenated to deoxygenated haemoglobin, and so the percentage of oxygen saturation.

The actual amount of haemoglobin present in the blood changes with altitude: the body increases the rate at which it manufactures haemoglobin-carrying red blood cells as a result of acclimatization to high altitudes. If you were placed from sea level on to the summit of Mount Everest, giving the body no chance to acclimatize, you would quickly die. Because air pressure drops as you climb to altitude, the force pushing oxygen through the membranes of the lungs is reduced. For this reason, less oxygen dissolves in the blood plasma running through the lungs, and this results in less oxygen being taken up by the red blood cells. To offset this, the body steps up its rate of manufacture of red blood cells. There are other, more subtle changes that take place in a body that is acclimatizing, but the increase in red blood cell production is the most important. While the extra red blood cells allow enough oxygen to be carried to where it is needed, they can actually be a problem, too. The extra volume of red blood cells thickens the blood, slowing the flow and increasing the risk of the blood clotting.

The process of acclimatization is initiated by small organs located in the neck, next to the carotid artery that conducts blood to the head. These organs, carotid and aortic bodies, contain clumps of nerve cells that respond to changes in the blood's pH (how acid or alkaline it is) as well as the concentration of dissolved oxygen. Blood's pH is related to the amount of carbon dioxide present – carbon dioxide gas dissolves in water (and therefore blood) to produce a solution that is slightly acidic. The function of the carotid and aortic bodies is not well understood, but they seem to initiate a chain of events that increases the blood's oxygen saturation, which helps to rid the body of carbon dioxide. You can think of these organs as hypoxia sensors. They are connected to a part of the brain called the medulla, one of the roles of which is to control breathing rate. Doctors sometimes administer to certain patients a mixture of oxygen and carbon dioxide – the carbon dioxide causes the medulla to increase breathing rate, so that more of the oxygen is taken in. The carotid bodies are also thought to release a substance that stimulates an increase in levels of a hormone called erythropoietin. It is an increase in this hormone – itself due to the release of yet another hormone by the kidneys – that causes the bone marrow to increase the rate at which it manufactures red blood cells. So when a climber first arrives at high altitude, and becomes hypoxic, his or her body responds first by increasing the breathing rate, and then by increasing the number of red blood cells in the blood. There is also some evidence of a thinning of the membranes of the alveoli in the lungs.

All these changes act to increase the potential of the blood to carry oxygen, to compensate for the reduction in oxygen in the atmosphere. People who live at high altitudes have higher red blood cell counts than those who live at lower altitudes. Strangely, this seems to change over time – almost as if a person's body becomes tired of being acclimatized twenty-four hours of every day. The 'chronic mountain sickness' that ensues is sometimes called Monge's disease, after the Peruvian doctor who identified the condition in the 1920s. It has been studied in a number of research projects, including one carried out on a population of Peruvian people who live in and around the highest city in the world, Cerro de Pasco, which is 4,340 metres (14,200 feet) above sea level. The people who had lived there the longest tended to suffer the most. Yaks and other animals that live at high altitude are born better able to cope with lower atmospheric pressure and density – they are adapted, not acclimatized, to high altitudes.

During the process of acclimatization, symptoms of mild and moderate acute mountain sickness – such as a throbbing headache, nausea and vomiting and debilitating fatigue – are common. These are largely due to the brain actually swelling inside the skull at high altitude. The swelling is caused by plasma fluid leaking out of blood vessels inside the head, and puts pressure on the brain, as well as displacing some of the cerebrospinal fluid – in which the brain is normally bathed – down into the spinal cord. This may explain some of the impairment in cognitive performance as well as the headaches. If the body does not fully acclimatize to each increase in elevation, for example, if it is not given enough time to do so, then a climber may suffer from more debilitating or even life-threatening problems. The most severe problems are caused by fluid leaking from capillaries into certain tissues of the body. When fluid – blood plasma with some red blood cells – leaks into a climber's lungs, the climber will develop a rasping and incessant cough, and the struggle for air will increase with each breath. This condition is known as high-altitude pulmonary oedema. Peter Hackett, the physiologist involved in the expedition, explains that 'the air sacs start to fill up ... the person starts coughing a pink frothy sputum, can't get any air at all; they go into cardiovascular collapse and die'.

Another life-threatening condition is high-altitude cerebral oedema, which is an extreme form of acute mountain sickness. In this distressing illness, where the fluid build-up in the brain has increased to dangerous levels, disorientation and general mental dysfunction can give way to psychotic behaviour and coma. Sometimes people hallucinate. Both cerebral and pulmonary oedema can be fatal if not treated quickly and appropriately. The ideal treatment is rapid descent by a few hundred metres to air with higher pressure and density. In situations where the patient is unable to walk or be transported easily, a clever but simple invention can save his or her life by simulating just such a rapid descent. This invention is the Gamow bag: a sealable, body-sized plastic bag, which acts like a portable emergency hyperbaric oxygen chamber. To simulate lower altitudes, the seriously hypoxic patient is sealed inside the bag, and a foot pump is used to increase the air pressure – and therefore the oxygen pressure – inside the bag. After an hour or two inside a Gamow bag, the patient is usually well enough to walk down to lower altitudes, where he or she can recover.

Move on up

After a few days of acclimatizing at Base Camp, the climbers set off up the Khumbu Icefall – the most treacherous part of the climb. This involved crossing crevasses on metal ladders and climbing steep walls of ice. They were heading for Camp I, which is at an altitude of 5,940 metres (19,500 feet). The icefall is filled with huge chunks of ice, each the size of a house, and these chunks can move without warning, sometimes taking climbers with them. On arrival at Camp I, the climbers measured their pulse and their oxygen saturation levels with the pulse oxymeter, and took the psychometric tests. The saturation levels were as expected for this altitude. David Breashears radioed the team at Base Camp and reported an oxygen saturation of

80 per cent and a pulse of about 78. In fact, as he was radioing and being filmed, he also reported 'test anxiety', which was causing his pulse to race up to 104. Test anxiety may not be the only thing that seemed to affect the results. Perhaps due to fatigue, David Carter gave the wrong answer to a true-or-false question, announcing that the statement 'Lion is a military title' was true. Even taking into account test anxiety and fatigue, the climbers did seem to be thinking more slowly, and their judgement seemed to be impaired.

More tests would have to be carried out, at various altitudes, to collect enough data to be able to come to any useful conclusions about reduction in blood oxygen and mental dysfunction. After a few days at Camp I, the climbers descended to the 'showers, oxygen, warmth and cotton clothing' at Base Camp, where they would recuperate before ascending again. On their way down, they were caught at a bottleneck, where climbers can descend only one at a time. Talking from the top of the Khumbu Icefall, Breashears joked: 'It's amazing – we're on Everest and we're waiting in line.'

The team were to spend more than two months on the mountain, gradually working their way up to the summit, taking time and care to acclimatize and rest between each stage. Their schedule is typical of expeditions to conquer Mount Everest:

UP from Base Camp to Camp I
DOWN from Camp I to Base Camp
UP from Base Camp to Camp I
UP from Camp I to Camp II
DOWN from Camp II to Base Camp
UP from Base Camp to Camp II
UP from Camp II to Camp III
DOWN to Base Camp
UP through Camps I, II, III, to Camp IV
UP to the summit.

The climbers could stop for a few days at Base Camp and at Camps I and II. But they could stay just two nights at Camp III and only overnight at Camp IV, which are in the 'death zone' where humans can be only transient visitors. The reason for this is that where the air is very thin, and oxygen intake is much lower than normal, a climber's body rapidly deteriorates, the muscles waste away and consume themselves just to survive. There is a maximum rate at which a person's heart can beat. This is generally well above the heart rate at rest, so there is scope for an increase in heart rate demanded by physical exertion. However, as we have seen, heart rate at rest increases with altitude, and this leaves less scope for an increase during exertion. Eventually, above about 7,920 metres (26,000 feet), the heart rate at rest becomes very close to the maximum heart rate. Acclimatization can offset this effect only slightly, and climbers without breathing apparatus are in great danger in the death zone. In fact, physician Peter Hackett explains that, in the death zone, 'acclimatization is essentially impossible'. Add to this the fact that, at this altitude, it is impossible for helicopters to reach stranded climbers because the air is so rarefied, and you can see why this is called the death zone. Breashears and his team were carrying cylinders containing compressed oxygen with face masks, for use at and just below the summit. A few people have climbed to the summit of Mount Everest without using supplemental oxygen, including Ed Viesturs on two occasions. The first people to do so were Reinhold Messner and Peter Habeler in 1978.

After their second ascent to Camp I, and the subsequent ascent to Camp II and descent to Base Camp, the climbers made their way up to Camps II and III, and then down to Base Camp again. At Base Camp, a sick Sherpa was being treated by the doctor of a Malaysian expedition. The Sherpa had been found very ill: according to the Malaysian doctor, he was 'ashen grey, breathless' and his oxygen saturation level was a dangerous 20 per cent. He was given pure oxygen, which boosted his oxygen saturation to 80 per cent, and, after spending two hours in a Gamow bag, he was well enough to be flown down to Kathmandu in a helicopter. Another Sherpa, found lying in the middle of the trail below Base Camp, was not so lucky. A Canadian doctor who attended him diagnosed him as suffering from extreme pulmonary oedema – he was 'drowning in his own secretions', and he died soon after he was discovered.

Breashears and his team prepared themselves for the final ascent, which they hoped would take them up to the summit. As they made their way up the Khumbu Icefall, they came across some human remains – the bones of a foot still in a climbing shoe. According to Howard Donner, 'this sort of stuff is spilling out all the time'. The climbers bypassed Camp I, pushed on up the Western Cwm, and stayed a few nights at Camp II, known as Advance Base Camp, at an altitude of 7,040 metres (23,100 feet). The climbers' oxygen saturation levels and pulse rates changed as you would expect with the increase in altitude. The psychometric tests, too, showed that the climbers' brains were taking longer to process information, and were prone to making more mistakes. Over the radio, Ed Viesturs hears the question: 'If Daphne walks twice as fast as Margaret, and they are the only two people in the race, who is most likely to finish last?' Viesturs hesitated a little longer than he would have done at sea level, but he answered correctly and confidently. By this stage of the expedition, David Carter had developed what he described as 'a real violent cough; it comes from deep within … my main concern is that when I get higher, the cough will get worse, and I'm worried about breaking a rib or vomiting or something'. He had conquered a head cold that had troubled him earlier on in the expedition, but his health was still a real worry. Despite this, he was determined to make it to the summit this time, after his failure to do so in 1991. From Camp II, at the bottom of the

Lhotse Face, the climbers made an arduous ascent up to Camp III, where they would stay for two days and nights before moving on towards Camp IV and the summit.

At Camp III – at an elevation of 7,500 metres (24,600 feet) – the pulse oxymeter readings showed that the high altitudes were putting the climbers under increasing physical stress. David Carter, in poor health, had a pulse of 140 beats per minute and an oxygen saturation level of just 60 per cent. As he was approaching Camp III, David Breashears asked him about how the climb was going. Carter replied, 'It's tiring, it's slow; you're winded, you're dehydrated, you're losing your voice, you're coughing; but the views make it worth it.' The psychometric tests at Camp III indicated that the climbers' brains were definitely beginning to slow down, and their confusion and lack of attention was evident. Ed Viesturs was asked to repeat the following sentence over the radio: 'The video camera captured the bank robber's daring daylight robbery of the First Avenue Bank.' He said, with breathless hesitation: 'The video camera captured the daring bank robber's robbery of the First National Bank.' When repeating similar sentences at lower altitudes, Viesturs had done much better than this, and without hesitation. Similarly, David Breashears was asked to repeat this sentence: 'The action of the brave cyclist kept the small boy from being hit by a ten-tonne truck.' His attempt was: 'The action of the brave cyclist ... um ... helped ... uh ... save the boy ... let's see, I know I have to repeat all I know ... prevent the boy being hit by the ten-tonne truck – oh shit.' The poor performance of the climbers' brains at this altitude – no doubt caused by a combination of hypoxia and fatigue – put them at risk of serious accident or death. Camp III is situated on a 45 degree slope of ice and snow and many climbers have died there as a result of just one poorly placed step.

After a night at Camp III, the climbers pushed on towards Camp IV, called the South Col, situated at the top of the Lhotse Face. The climbers had taken two months to reach this point. Breathing supplemental oxygen through a mouthpiece attached to the nozzle of a canister in their rucksacks, each climber's oxymeter reading increased. But the climbers were still out of breath as they bravely continued with the psychometric tests. Their performance was slower still, and they made more errors than before in repeating sentences. Over the radio from Base Camp, Dr Howard Donner asked David Carter to repeat the following: 'Ed lived by the river for twenty years and only twice before in all those years had it been this high.' Carter replied breathlessly, and with a few errors: 'Ed lived by the river for twenty years and this was the first time it had ever been this high.'

Climbers at this stage of the ascent of Mount Everest, with or without supplemental oxygen, are extremely tired, and it is exhausting just gasping for breath. After just half a night at Camp IV, Breashears and his team set off for the summit. Peter Hackett, expedition physiologist, explained the magnitude of this task: 'When one considers the condition that a climber is in at the South Col on summit day, it's really amazing that they can reach the summit at all. First of all, there hasn't been sleep for usually a couple of nights; there hasn't been enough to eat or drink; even if they've been on oxygen, it's still been very uncomfortable to breathe. The mucous membranes are all dried out – there's always a sore throat, there's always a cough, there's often a headache. It takes a tremendous amount of will to keep going in these conditions.'

Peak performance

The team decided to make their move for the summit in the late evening, and climb during the night. This was so that they would not get caught up with other climbers making the same journey. So at ten o'clock on the evening of 22 May, the team left Camp IV, heading for the summit. The final stages of the climb involved a difficult trek along the treacherous, knife-edge, south-east ridge that rises fewer than a hundred metres (300 feet), to a point just beneath the summit. To get to the summit, the climbers had to conquer one more hurdle – the Hillary Step, a 12-metre (40-foot) face of rock and ice. This they did and, exhausted but jubilant, every member of the team made it to the summit at around six o'clock in the morning. Breashears was the first to pull himself up on to the summit itself, and he erected the Tibetan flag in the snow. The atmospheric pressure at the summit is about thirty-four per cent of the atmospheric pressure at sea level – this is about as high as people can go without supplemental oxygen or being in a pressurized capsule, such as an aeroplane fuselage. The views from this, the highest point on Earth, were incredible.

David Breashears announced on the radio, to Howard Donner at Base Camp, that he was 'on top of the world', and he and Ed Viesturs took their final physiological and psychometric tests of the expedition. Their oxygen saturation levels were between 70 and 80 per cent – higher than they had been for much of the expedition because of the pure oxygen they had been breathing. Donner asked Breashears to repeat the sentence 'Mike walked around the block three times until he had the nerve to knock on Carol's door.' Even on the top of Mount Everest, after the weeks of physical and mental effort that it took to get there, Breashears answered with but one error: he said '... walk on Carol's door'. Ed Viesturs was asked: 'A man who is an engineer came to the store where Alice worked to buy pastries; who bought pastries?' After a long, anguished hesitation, he replied: 'The man ... Jack ... the engineer.' He giggled, clearly confused.

After his tests, Breashears described to Donner what he had seen as he passed the site of the previous year's tragedy, at the Hillary Step. He explained, 'All the bodies that were there last year were covered, but unfortunately we did pass one body right on the fixed rope; it only makes me question my sanity, why I climbed this mountain again, because it is dangerous and cold.' David Carter could not take the psychometric tests at the summit because he had lost his voice. The climbers left the summit and, after five hours of more hard work, made it down to Camp IV. Many of the 150 or so people who have died on Mount Everest have perished on their way down from the summit – the relief of making it to the top causes many climbers to lose concentration.

Back at Camp IV, Carter's condition became worse still. His oxygen saturation was a healthy 93 per cent, with the supplemental oxygen, but he could not breathe at all well and was suffering badly. Ed Viesturs attempted to take him down to much lower altitudes, but because of Carter's condition the two had to stop every few metres so that Carter could catch his breath. In fact, they made it only as far as Camp III. That evening, Viesturs made an emergency call down to Base Camp, shouting, 'David's dying!' Dr Donner was on hand to help him to try to save Carter's life. Carter, already dangerously short of breath, was choking on something that he had coughed up. Viesturs performed the Heimlich manoeuvre several times on him. This involves squeezing the patient hard, from behind, around the abdomen, forcing a sudden burst of air up the windpipe to dislodge any blockage. It saved Carter's life. In the morning, Carter was a lot better, and he was able to make it down the mountain to Base Camp.

All safely back at Base Camp, the climbers and the medical and scientific team were soon on their way back home. Ten days later, the team met back in Seattle, at the University of Washington, to assess the pulse oxymeter measurements and the results of the psychometric tests. The climbers also went back into the MRI scanner, so that any slight damage to the brain or change in brain size during the mission might be detected by comparing the post-expedition scans with those taken before it. As expected, the oxygen saturation levels were generally lower at higher altitudes, apart from when supplemental oxygen was used. It was interesting to note that David Carter's oxygen saturation levels were consistently lower than those of the other climbers – this presumably had something to do with his sickness on the mountain. The results of the psychometric tests also seemed to be dependent on oxygen levels in the climbers' blood, as you would expect. The results of the MRI scans were less clear – more analysis and further tests will need to be done to ascertain whether prolonged reduction in blood oxygen due to altitude leads to any temporary or permanent brain damage. The only damage the MRI scans picked up were, according to Dr Hackett, 'a very mild atrophy in the brain of Ed Viesturs, who was the one that had climbed many times to high altitude without supplemental oxygen. And what we'd like to do is follow him over a longer period of time to see if this is something that might actually progress with his high-altitude career.' On reviewing the psychometric test results, which illustrated the slowing of mental functioning, the expedition's psychometrist, Gail Rosenbaum, told the team: 'The question we ask is, "What happens if you are in an emergency situation – are you able to think quickly and clearly about what you need to do to survive?"'

As more and more people want to scale the heights of the world's great mountains, it becomes ever more important that scientists and mountaineers understand the effects of hypoxia. Eight people died in that single incident in 1996, the year before Breashears and his team carried out the expedition detailed above. And as the 1997 expedition was ending, there was a similar tragedy on the other side of the mountain. Shortly after the expedition was over, in a radio interview on WGBH, the radio station that followed the expedition, David Breashears spoke about the worries he had about the increasing numbers of people climbing Mount Everest. 'And despite what happened last year, not a lot of lessons have been learned. People will continue to come here with great hopes and dreams, and some of them will make it and some of them will die. And that's the nature of climbing on the highest mountain in the world.'

LIES AND DELUSIONS
...searching for the self...

So far, we have looked at some of the remarkable discoveries being made in the quest to understand the brain and how it works. One of the most powerful tools in this quest is the study of what happens when something goes wrong. This last chapter focuses on damage sustained by the cerebrum, the most prominent and the most complex part of the brain. The walnut-shaped cerebrum – which consists of two large hemispheres – takes up most of the volume and most of the mass of the brain. It is thought to be responsible for some of the higher brain functions, so it will come as no surprise that damage to the cerebrum will cause the loss of some of our most remarkable behaviours or abilities. We saw in the first chapter 'Mind Readers' how damage to the orbito-frontal cortex can cause a dramatic shift in a person's personality – changing a calm, thoughtful and sensitive person into a selfish, bad-tempered bore. The cases described in this last chapter explore other changes that can occur in an individual's beliefs, behaviour, physical abilities or perception as a result of damage to the cerebrum. The resulting neurological disorders are fascinating, though sometimes disturbing, and they can be very revealing about how the undamaged cerebrum works. The study of the effects of damage to the cerebrum may also help to realize one of the ambitions of the study of the brain: to work out how your brain creates a sense of your 'self'.

Convoluted story

The role of the cerebrum in producing a sense of self was illustrated in 'Phantom Brains', where we discovered that there is a sensory map of the body on the outer surface of the cerebrum, the cortex. The deep wrinkles of this incredibly complex sheet of brain tissue mean that it can have a surface area almost as large as a pillowcase and still fit around a brain not much larger than a fist. There are many millions of neurones in the cortex, connected by literally thousands of kilometres of fibres. This amazing place is alive with waves of electricity coursing along the fibres that interconnect the neurones. It is here that much of our perception and learning take place, and it seems that it is here that we initiate the conscious actions that make up our behaviour.

Just what kind of disruption a person suffers to his or her mental faculties as a result of damage to the cerebrum depends upon where the damage is sustained, and what type of cortex is damaged. There are three different types of cortex: sensory, motor and association. The last of these generally lies between areas of the other two, and there is a flow of information – from the sensory, through the association, to the motor cortex. The connections between the neurones in all three types of cortex change over time, according to the sensations received and the experiences gained by the person whose brain they inhabit. But it is areas of association cortex that seem to hold the bulk of our memories of past experience, which are used to produce the appropriate action for particular sensory input. The recognition of familiar objects, decisions about what to say, understanding spoken words and producing precise, skilled movements are all carried out in areas of association cortex.

The two hemispheres of the cerebrum are close together but separate. There is a vertical cleft that extends down between the hemispheres, again just like a walnut. As well as the many small furrows shaped by the wrinkles in the cortex, there are two much deeper furrows that conveniently divide each hemisphere into four lobes. These are the frontal lobes found behind the forehead; the parietal lobes, beneath the top of the head; the occipital lobes, right at the back of the cerebrum; and the temporal lobes, situated inside the parts of the skull where the ears are.

Studies of patients with damage to their brains are useful; but such studies are not the only way of gathering an understanding of how the brain works. This is an important point: when part of the brain is damaged, the resulting behaviour of the patient is actually more a reflection of the capabilities of the remaining parts of the brain than of the damaged part itself. Knowledge about the connections between different parts of the brain, its biochemistry and the behaviour of individual neurones is just as useful in the quest to understand this complex organ. However, in the early days of neurophysiology, matching damage in particular areas of the cortex to brain dysfunction was the main method available.

The first person to link a brain function with a particular area of the cortex was a French surgeon, Pierre-Paul Broca, in 1861. Broca studied the strange speech problems of one of his patients, a man known as 'Tan-tan' because that was all he could say. This kind of problem is an example of aphasia, the loss of the ability to use or understand words. In a post-mortem examination of Tan-tan's brain, Broca discovered damage localized to part of the patient's cortex in the frontal lobe of the left cerebral hemisphere. Broca followed up this case by carrying out a further eight post-mortems on patients who had suffered from similar aphasias. The area of the cortex damaged in these patients, towards the front of the brain above the temples, is now called Broca's area. A little more than a decade after Broca made his discovery, the German neurologist Carl Wernicke made a similar one – this time locating the area of the cortex that seemed to be responsible for understanding the meanings of words. Patients suffering from Wernicke's aphasia are able to speak fluently and even construct sentences using correct grammar – but what they say has no meaning, and they have trouble understanding what is said to them. Wernicke's area is further back in the brain, in the left parietal lobe. As you might expect, there are large bundles of nerve fibres connecting Broca's area with Wernicke's area.

Since the days of Broca and Wernicke, thousands more detailed accounts of strange brain disorders, together with examinations of abnormalities in the brain, have continued to provide clues to the functions of most of the regions of the cortex. The range of dysfunctions is almost as diverse – and equally as mind-boggling – as the range of abilities that the normal human brain possesses. Neurology has devised a comprehensive list of names for the various disorders exhibited by patients with damage to the cortex. For example, in addition to aphasia there is alexia (loss of the ability to read); apraxia (loss of the ability to perform complex tasks); agraphia (loss of the ability to write); agnosia (loss of the ability to recognize things or people). Each of these is subdivided according to the specific nature of the loss of ability: for example, auditory agnosia is the inability to recognize sounds, while tactile agnosia is the inability to recognize objects by touch.

The damage causing disorders such as aphasia and agnosia is normally the result of injury or disease. Damage to the cortex of a boxer is a gradual accumulation over many years, and can lead to a general slowing of mental function or specific problems such as those with speech. Road traffic accidents are the most common cause of injury to the cortex. Pedestrians who are knocked down often suffer a deceleration injury, as their head slams against the road. Drivers who are involved in collisions and who are not wearing seat belts may suffer a similar injury as their heads smash against the windscreen. The physical damage produced by a deceleration injury or a violent blow to the head can cause bruising or laceration in the tissue of the cortex, or haemorrhaging inside the skull. A haemorrhage may be caused by blood escaping from arteries, and therefore not reaching the tissues for which it was intended; this can lead to the death of neurones in the cortex. Haemorrhages can also exert physical pressure on the cortex, and this too can cause the death of neurones. Among the afflictions that cause the death of brain tissue are Alzheimer's disease and Creutzfeldt–Jakob Disease (CJD); another is stroke, which is by far the most common. While Alzheimer's disease and CJD generally cause a gradual but widespread reduction in brain function – because they cause slow deterioration across the whole brain – strokes often cause more localized damage. A stroke involves the loss of blood normally due to blockage of one artery supplying the brain, and can lead to sudden and devastating paralysis or loss of memory, or in some cases more specific disorders such as those listed above. Whatever the cause of brain damage, that damage is known as a lesion.

Watching the unseen

One of the strangest things that can happen to a person's sense of the world as a result of a lesion to a specific region of the cerebrum is a condition known as 'blindsight'. Patients with blindsight can correctly 'guess' in which direction an object is moving, or unconsciously grab a moving object, even though they cannot actually see it. Blindsight patients are typically able to put an envelope through a letterbox in front of them without a second thought, even though they are not consciously aware of the letterbox. Most people with this odd affliction are only blind in part of their 'visual field' – typically one half. Such a person looking at the centre of this book would be able to see, say, the right-hand page but not the left.

The term 'blindsight' was coined by psychologist Lawrence Weiskrantz, who pioneered the study of the disorder at Oxford University during the 1970s. At the time, many researchers believed that it was simply due to weakened eyesight. Some neurologists thought that blindsight patients might be making up their remarkable ability. But careful observation of eye movements and monitoring of pupil dilation showed that blindsight patients really are blind in the normal sense of the word.

Professor Colin Blakemore, also at Oxford University, is a neurophysiologist who includes blindsight in the range of brain functions and dysfunctions that he studies. One of the blindsight patients he studies is Graham, who suffered injury to part of his cortex in a road accident more than thirty years ago, when he was eight years old. During careful tests of his condition, Graham sits in front of a desktop computer. The monitor screen is divided into two regions: white on the left of the screen and grey on the right. When Graham gazes at a grey dot just inside the white portion of the screen, the border of his blind field of vision lies at the border between the white and grey areas on the screen. He can see the white side of the screen on the left, just as any sighted person can, but he is blind to the grey side of the screen, on the right. So when Blakemore holds his hand in front of the grey part of the screen, Graham does not see it. But as soon as Blakemore moves his hand up and down, Graham responds, saying, 'You are moving it up and down.' Graham still does not actually see the hand, but part of his brain somehow registers the movement. As Graham continues to gaze at the grey dot on the screen, a series of black squares appears in the right-hand, grey portion of the monitor screen. Graham cannot see them. Each one moves off – up, down or to the right – soon after it appears, and Graham has to guess which way they have moved. He guesses right every time.

Blakemore explains why studies of blindsight are helping to uncover the way vision works: 'If there is one thing that this phenomenon of blindsight teaches us, it is that vision is not entirely seeing; that there can be a disconnection between the capacity to respond to visual information and the act of being visually aware.'

How can we explain the strange phenomenon of blind-sight? The current theory involves the fact that sensory input from the eyes travels along two separate pathways in the brain. It seems that one of these pathways allows us to be conscious of what we see, while the other provides our essential but unconscious visual functions, such as the ability to follow moving targets. Input to the eyes is generated when light falls on a layered sheet of cells at the back of the eye – the retina. Cells in one of the layers are sensitive to light, and stimulate the nerve endings of the optic nerve. Each eye collects information from both sides of the visual field – you can still see the whole of this book when you close one eye (assuming you are a sighted person with two eyes). A few centimetres behind the bridge of the nose is a point at which the optic nerve from each eye splits in two. This point is called the optic chiasma; on leaving it, the nerves from the left side of the visual field are separate from those that come from the right side. The bundle of nerve fibres from each side of the visual field now goes along the two separate pathways.

One of the two main pathways leads first to the thalamus, the way station for nearly all sensory information to the brain. One small part of each thalamus – called the lateral geniculate nucleus – is a relay station for visual information from the optic nerves. The information is routed from the thalami to the 'primary visual cortex' in the occipital lobes, at the backs of the two cerebral hemispheres. Just as there is a sensory map of the body – half of it in the cortex of each parietal lobe – the two halves of the visual field are 'mapped out' in the visual cortex. Visual signals from the left side end up at the right occipital lobe and vice versa. The primary visual cortex is connected to many other regions of the cerebrum. Damage to just a tiny part of a person's visual cortex means that that person will be blind in

the corresponding part of his or her visual field. It was damage to Graham's left occipital lobe that left him blind in the
right half of his visual field.

This first visual pathway – from the eyes through the
thalamus to the visual cortex – is more important in
humans and most other primates, such as chimpanzees,
than in dogs and cats. A dog, a cat, or any other animal less
sophisticated than humans has a smaller cerebrum and so
this pathway is not as important. This seems to tie in with
observations of the behaviour of animals that see their
reflections in mirrors. Whether or not an animal recognizes
itself in a mirror is the classic test for visual self-awareness.
It was devised in 1969 by Professor Gordon Gallup Junior,
then at Washington State University. Most animals react as
if they are looking at another animal when confronted with
their reflection. But humans (from about eighteen months
old) and chimpanzees and orang-utans (from adolescence)
do recognize themselves. Chimpanzees and orang-utans
that have had some experience of mirrors will, for example,
notice a mark on the face in the mirror and immediately
reach up to their own face to investigate. Reptiles have vir-
tually no cerebrum, and we can assume that they are not
really conscious of what they see in the same way. Instead,
they rely only on automatic, instinctive reactions to visual
information. This information is supplied by the second
visual pathway, which developed in ancient evolutionary
history: it is common to all mammals, amphibians, birds
and reptiles. It passes directly from the optic nerve to a
structure at the top of the brain stem called the superior colliculus. In animals with little or no cerebrum, this visual
pathway ends in the superior colliculus; in humans and the
higher primates, it continues to the parietal lobes. The
superior colliculus initiates automatic movements that
direct an animal's vision towards an object of interest – a
predator or a potential meal, for example. The rapid,
unconscious movements that direct your eyes are called

saccades, and are initiated by the superior colliculus itself, just as in the reptiles and other animals. But the signals carried along this pathway, which arrive in the parietal lobes, are thought to give a sense of space, directing attention consciously to objects in the visual field.

In Graham's brain, the pathway that leads from the retinas of the eyes to the superior colliculus is intact. For this reason, Graham can react unconsciously to objects moving in the blind part of his visual field. The damage to his visual cortex – the end of the other visual pathway – means that he is not aware of the objects. This explains Graham's blindsight. In reptiles, such as lizards, blindsight is normal because they have no visual cortex. Graham explains that – in half of his visual field at least – he and a lizard are 'distinct cousins'.

Although most of us do not suffer from blindsight, we all benefit from the automatic behaviour of the 'older' pathway involved in this strange condition. For example, if you are driving, your consciousness may be engaged in talking to someone next to you or listening to music – many of the routine aspects of driving are being carried out subconsciously, using the primitive visual pathway. It would seem from the study of blindsight, then, that there is an unconscious aspect of vision. This seems to be true in fully sighted people as well as those with blindsight. People who can see normally do not become aware of these unconscious factors but, in blindsight patients, there is no conscious aspect of vision to mask the unconscious behaviour. This is one of many clues that the cortex is heavily involved in producing consciousness.

One-sided view
In blindsight, the evolutionarily more recent visual pathway – which allows us to be conscious of what we see – is damaged; the older pathway – which initiates automatic, unconscious, responses – is intact. What would happen if

this situation were reversed? In other words, what would happen if a person sustained damage to the older pathway, while the newer pathway remained intact? Would we then have the opposite of blindsight? Professor Vilayanur Ramachandran, Director of the Center for Brain Cognition at the University of California, San Diego, (whose research on the phantom-limb phenomenon was discussed in 'Phantom Brains'.) has been very active in recent years in attempting to explain some of the strange syndromes associated with damage to the cortex, including blindsight. He suggests that patients who suffer a stroke focused in the right parietal lobe experience something like the opposite of blindsight.

As described above, areas of the parietal lobes are the end point of the older visual pathway, and the parietal lobes seem to be involved in spatial awareness and in tracking moving objects. It has been shown, for example, that neurones in the parietal lobes become active when an object enters the visual field. So you might expect people who have suffered damage to the older visual pathway, in the parietal lobe, to be visually aware of the world but unable to carry out the unconscious tracking of moving objects. And you would be right: such patients are said to suffer from 'visual neglect'. They may also suffer disruption to their spatial awareness. Asking one visual-neglect patient, Bill, to track his finger as it moves horizontally in front of his face, Ramachandran demonstrates this idea. Bill suffered a stroke in his right parietal lobe, and the left side of his body is largely paralysed. His head and neck are skewed to the right – he describes his upper body as being 'twisted like a pretzel'. Bill's head and eyes remain stationary as Ramachandran's finger moves in front of him, although he can correctly describe the motion and knows that it is the professor's finger. Ramachandran explains that Bill 'can no longer point to something on the left side of the world ... and can no longer orient to what's going on to the left; he's not blind – his visual cortex is still normal'. Another patient suffering from visual neglect is Peggy, who compares her condition to 'like just before you faint: everything disappears'. Her visual neglect becomes clear when she tries to draw: copying a four-pointed star, she draws only three points, leaving out the one on the left. Similarly, drawing daisies, she includes the correct number of petals, but all of them are squashed awkwardly on to the right-hand side of the stalk. 'I've done it on all of them!' she exclaims, looking at her drawings after she has finished.

One way of investigating the extent of visual neglect is to ask patients to use a mirror to bring the missing part of the visual field – left of the patient – into view. You might expect patients suffering from neglect to turn to their left when they see an object of interest in the mirror. This seems reasonable, because these patients have not lost their mind – they are still aware of how things work, including mirrors. Ramachandran holds a mirror on Bill's right and asks him to reach for a set of keys held to Bill's left, but which appear in the mirror to the right. Surprisingly perhaps, Bill attempts to reach into the mirror, however much he tries to concentrate, and despite the fact that he is fully aware that the keys he can see are part of a mirror image. Ramachandran says that the job of working out the relationship between a real object and its mirror image is the sort of process carried out by the parietal lobe, and this explains why Bill simply cannot reach for the real keys. He says that it is as if Bill is saying to himself 'on my planet, left does not exist'. Interestingly, when the same experiment is carried out with the mirror in front of Bill's face, and the keys held behind his head, Bill is able to reach behind him to grasp the keys. In this case, he makes use of the spatial awareness of his undamaged, left parietal lobe to achieve this task.

In some patients with right parietal lobe damage, neglect is so extreme that not only do their brains deny the existence of space to their left, they may even deny the existence of the left side of their own bodies. One patient studied by Professor Ramachandran, a Mrs Sinclair, claimed that she was being shown her husband's hand – 'I've been living with him for twenty-seven years, I know his hand' – when actually it was her own, paralysed, hand that was being held up. An extension of this, and even more bizarre, is a disorder known as anosagnosia, also found in people with right parietal lobe damage. People with anosagnosia lie – even to themselves – about their paralysis or other conditions that result from their brain damage. These other conditions, well documented but not completely understood, include inability to draw, to dress or to construct things. People with anosagnosia do not deny their symptoms simply because they are ashamed of them – other patients with damage to their brains do not behave in this way. Mrs Sinclair showed signs of anosagnosia: during each of Professor Ramachandran's first few visits, she said that she could use the paralysed hand. In one task used to test patients with anosagnosia, they are asked to touch a doctor's nose with a finger of their paralysed left hand. Of course, they cannot direct their paralysed arm towards the doctor's nose. Rather than explaining that their left arm is paralysed, most anosagnosic patients will make up excuses for their arm's inactivity. When Ramachandran asks Bill to attempt the test, Bill explains that he is 'calling up his arm ... explaining to it what to do ... it's tired'. Some patients actually claim that they are touching the doctor's nose with their hand.

Another revealing test of the nature of this strange disorder is asking a patient with anosagnosia to clap. Bill makes the normal motions of clapping with his right hand, fooling himself that the other hand is doing the same. But his good hand ends up hitting the air, and then his chest, as the paralysed arm lies motionless on his lap. Bill seems to believe that he is clapping normally. Anosagnosia was first described nearly a hundred years ago by French neurologist Joseph Babinski, one of the pioneers of experimental neurology. But only now are neurologists and neurophysiologists discovering how the symptoms might relate to damage to the right parietal lobe.

Lesions to either parietal lobe can lead to a number of different symptoms, depending on where the damage is sustained. The sensory map on the cortex is located on the parietal lobe, and damage to that area in either hemisphere leads to a loss of sensation in part of the opposite side of the body. Damage to the motor areas of a person's parietal lobes results in that person being unable to carry out skilled movements – apraxia. When other areas of the parietal lobe are damaged, patients may suffer from agnosia (inability to recognize familiar objects). There are several different types of agnosia, again depending on where in the parietal lobe, and in which parietal lobe, the lesion occurs. Lesions to areas of the left parietal lobe result in tactile agnosia – the loss of ability to recognize objects by touch. Anosagnosia is caused only by damage to the right parietal lobe. The fact that the nature of a neurological disorder depends upon which cerebral hemisphere is damaged has been known since the time of Broca and Wernicke, mentioned above. Both types of aphasia that they described were caused by damage to the left side of the brain.

Which is right?
In 1874 Wernicke published a book in which he described various deficits in cognitive function caused by damage to specific areas of the cortex. As part of his descriptions, he claimed that certain abilities are found in only one of the cerebral hemispheres. Some of the earliest attempts to work out which parts of the cortex are responsible for which brain functions were carried out by German researchers Gustav Fritsch and Eduard Hitzig in the 1860s. Hitzig began this process while working in a military hospital, taking

advantage of patients whose skulls had been damaged in battle: he stimulated exposed areas of the cortex using wires connected to a battery. Around 1870 Fritsch and Hitzig found, in experiments on dogs, that electrical stimulation of one cerebral hemisphere produced movement in the opposite side of the body.

Signals to and from the left side of the body are carried by nerve bundles separate from those to and from the right side of the body. Above the top of the spinal cord, in the brainstem, the nerve bundles to and from the rest of the body cross over. Nerves to and from the eyes, ears, mouth and the rest of the head also cross over in this way. This explains why the visual map in the left occipital lobe receives signals from the right side of the visual field, and vice versa, as we saw in the discussion of blindsight, above. Similarly, the two sensory maps of the body – one on each parietal lobe – correspond to the opposite sides of the body. There are similar maps of the body on the motor cortex of the frontal lobes. Stimulating the area on this map corresponding to a finger will cause a person's finger to twitch. As with Fritsch and Hitzig's dog, the map on the cortex of the left frontal lobe corresponds to the right side of the body. Similarly, signals from the left ear arrive in the auditory (sensory) cortex of the right hemisphere.

Startling evidence of the differing abilities of the two cerebral hemispheres was found in experiments carried out by Roger Sperry and his colleagues at the California Institute of Technology, highlighting important differences between the two sides. The experiments involved surgically cutting through the corpus callosum – the dense bridge of nerve fibres that acts as the main pathway for signals between the two hemispheres. This resulted in 'split-brain' patients, whose two isolated cerebral hemispheres were unable to communicate with each other. The experiments were a desperate attempt to cure severe epilepsy. After patients recovered from these operations, they seemed to have all the faculties of people whose cerebral hemispheres have not been separated. However, further study showed that there were some important differences: the two sides of the brain seemed able to act independently, unaware of each other. For example, while the left hand of a 'split-brain' patient was buttoning a shirt, his right hand was busy unbuttoning it. More importantly, careful studies of split-brain patients revealed differences in function between the two hemispheres. So, for example, they found it easier to identify objects held in the right hand – interpreted by the left hemisphere – than in the left; they could copy drawings better with their left hand than their right, even if they were right-handed.

In a more recent split-brain experiment, conducted by Michael Gazzanioa at Cornell University in New York State, a split-brain patient was shown written commands in only one half of the visual field at a time. When the patient was shown the word 'laugh' in the left visual field (linked to the right hemisphere), he laughed but could not explain why. In fact, he made up reasons why he may have laughed, using his left hemisphere, which is more specialized to deal with language. The left hemisphere seems to have observed the laughter, and attempted to invent a story that would account for it.

The results of these and several other studies of split-brain patients have helped to show that the two hemispheres approach tasks differently. The left hemisphere is more concerned with logic, mathematical calculation and language than the right. The right hemisphere is more concerned with recognizing shapes and faces and appreciating music and art; it works holistically, analysing form and other visual-spatial aspects. One of the hemispheres is normally dominant – this explains handedness. If a person's left hemisphere is dominant, that person will be right-handed, and vice versa. Some people suggest that for this reason left-handed people are more likely to be creative, while right-handed people are more likely to think logically and have better language skills. There is some evidence to back up this idea, but it is by no means a hard and fast rule.

The different specialisms of the two cerebral hemispheres might help to explain the self-deceit involved in anosagnosia. Bill, whose anosagnosia made him fail to acknowledge his left-side paralysis, had suffered damage to his right parietal lobe. Anosagnosia is not found in patients with damage to the left parietal lobe. Professor Ramachandran has a theory that might help to explain this one-sided nature of anosagnosia. This involves the concept of the ego, first proposed by Sigmund Freud in the first two decades of the twentieth century.

Pleasing your self

Your senses provide information about the world around you – outside your body – but the information is put together inside your brain. It is there inside your brain that the information is interpreted and, more importantly, experienced. Your brain somehow constructs a feeling of yourself in the world. This sense of self is clearly an important part of consciousness, and is what Freud defined as the 'ego'. Consciousness itself is simply awareness. You can be conscious of a sound, an idea or the presence of a person, for example. Consciousness is elusive – modern neuropsychologists really have little idea how electrical signals in the brain can produce such a rich and ethereal experience. Until a decade or so ago, it was believed that consciousness is produced by the cortex, since that part of the brain is the most complex. The cortex clearly does play an important role in consciousness. Patients with blindsight are unaware of objects in the right visual field because of damage to their visual cortex, but can still react unconsciously to the things they 'see', for example. Research carried out using fMRI (functional magnetic resonance imaging) has confirmed that when blindsight patients react subconsciously to objects moving across their visual field, the superior colliculus – at the top of the brainstem, and not in the cortex – are active. However, most neuroscientists today tend to think that the cortex supplies the information – the thought processes and the ego – for other parts of the brain to be conscious of. While the cortex may not produce consciousness, what is known about it suggests that it is important in the creation of the ego, the self-image. The cortex is the destination for the incoming information, and it is the cortex that produces the 'higher' functioning of the brain. This includes speech, motor skills, memories and the recognition of objects, for example – all essential elements of our sense of self.

Ramachandran's theory of cortical remapping (explained in 'Phantom Brains') provides evidence that the cortex produces a 'body image', which seems like an important part of the self. When a person loses, say, a hand, he or she also loses sensory input from the hand to the relevant part of the sensory map on the cortex. Sensory input from different parts of the body – those that lie adjacent to the hand on the map – arrive at that part of the map previously associated with the hand. This has the strange consequence that a left-arm amputee will feel sensations in his or her non-existent (phantom) hand when touched on the cheek. The cortex seems to hold the blueprint for the body image, and when signals from the cheek arrive at the part of the cortex normally reserved for the hand, other parts of the brain become conscious of the hand. Historically, the first study to indicate that the cerebrum is important in producing conscious actions was carried out by the German physiologist Friedrich Goltz. In 1892 he found that dogs whose cerebrums had been removed lost all their abilities except their reflexes.

So how does the self – the ego – come into the behaviour of anosagnosic patients, who delude themselves about their left-arm paralysis? Ramachandran proposes that the ego might be produced by the left side of the brain, while the right brain includes a 'devil's advocate', which constantly checks to see if the self fits with the information received about the world. In a person whose brain is not damaged, but who has a paralysed arm, the ego may assert that the arm is not paralysed. But the right brain would be there to force the left brain to re-evaluate the ego. If the relevant part of the right brain is damaged, this devil's advocate would no longer function, enabling the left brain to construct the ego unchecked. In other words, once it has constructed the 'self', the brain seems to be prepared to lie to itself if the incoming information does not correspond to the self-image.

There is evidence that the brain does indeed work in this way, making up stories to account for what it perceives. In a famous study conducted at the University of California at San Francisco, brain researcher Benjamin Libet investigated people's awareness of their own will to cause their body to move. Before someone makes an apparently voluntary movement, such as flexing their wrist, a voltage called the readiness potential sweeps across the scalp. You might assume that the readiness potential is a result of a conscious decision to produce the movement. Libet asked his experimental subjects to flex their wrist or fingers whenever they felt they wanted to, and to declare that urge as soon as they were aware of it. He found that the awareness lagged behind the readiness potential by a consistent amount of time – about 0.4 seconds. You might think that this delay is simply the time it takes for a person to communicate the desire. But many other researchers have found similar results, which seem to suggest that consciousness really is a consequence of the unconscious behaviour of our brains, rather than a deciding factor or guiding light in how we should behave.

This calls into question the existence of free will – that ability we all seem to have to make decisions about our actions. As we live our lives day to day, we tend to assume that we make our own decisions about how we behave, or at least that we can do so whenever we want to. If someone asks you whether you want a cup of coffee, you think about it, make a decision and act upon that decision – you seem to have free will. However, some neuropsychologists believe that the brain reacts automatically in any situation, and that the mind works out what went on, making up reasons for behaviour shortly after the fact. According to this view, we are machines – automatons, behaving without conscious control. But at the same time, we are our own social commentators, supplying ourselves with reasons why we behave in the way we do – as if the mind is constantly looking for reasons why. Consciousness still has a role in this picture of behaviour: by monitoring your actions it can work out whether what happened was the best course of action in the circumstances, and learn from it. If this picture of consciousness – as an afterthought – is correct, it may explain why anosagnosic patients are able to lie to themselves. Ramachandran's theory suggests that the accounts of what is happening are produced largely in the left hemisphere and checked mainly by the right.

Ramachandran compares his suggested combination of ego and devil's advocate in his theory with the way that science arrives at its understanding of the world. The current theories at any time define the scientific view of the world. So, for example, physicists of the nineteenth century believed that time ran constantly and lengths were unchanging. Evidence to the contrary came from classic experiments during the 1880s, and from inconsistencies in the theories of electricity and magnetism. Physicists attempted to absorb these inconsistencies into their world view, trying to preserve stability in their theories, which had served them well until then. Albert Einstein's theories of relativity, the first of which he published in 1905, presented a new framework that explained the inconsistencies in the previous theory. Suddenly, the physicists' world view underwent a dramatic change – what philosophers call a paradigm shift. It is important that scientists work in this way: if they abandon their accepted theories whenever an inconsistency crops up, there would be no stability, no basis from which to move on. Ramachandran believes that in the brain, the ego in the left hemisphere is the stable sense of self, like the scientists' world view. The devil's advocate in the right hemisphere picks up on inconsistencies between the ego and the information it receives about the world or the body. It alerts the ego to the inconsistencies, so that it can undergo a paradigm shift.

So, according to Ramachandran, the brains of anosagnosic patients are able to deceive themselves about the state of the body they inhabit because their devil's advocate is no longer present. Freud believed that the ego was able to deceive the mind for the sake of its own stability, in just this way – until pressures on the ego became too much to bear and it would have to change. He suggested that the ego would use humour and self-deceit in defence of its own stability, and Ramachandran says that the kind of denial observed in anosagnosic patients is often tinged with a sense of humour or irony. It is as if the brain knows the truth but attempts to fool itself and other people. And indeed, the fact that the brain knows the truth about its body's condition is brought to light by a remarkable experiment on anosagnosic patients. When researchers trickle cold water into a patient's left ear, the delusion is broken – the patient is able to acknowledge their disability. Denial returns again after a few hours, and the patient cannot even recall being conscious of their paralysis. Cold water in the ear causes the brain to enter into a state something like dream-laden sleep: the eyes flicker rapidly as they do during the REM (rapid eye movement) phase of sleep, in which people dream. It is often in dreams that subconscious information, at other times suppressed, comes to the surface.

According to Ramachandran, the dreamlike state induced by the cold water allows the repressed knowledge of the paralysis to come to the surface.

Deceit is a fascinating aspect of human behaviour. Just why we have the ability to lie to each other and ourselves we may never know, though much thought has been given to it. Many evolutionary biologists consider deceit an important faculty in the animal world: it can be a crucial survival technique, and probably therefore evolved as part of animal behaviour. One such evolutionary biologist is Robert Trivers, one of the major figures in the world of sociobiology – also called evolutionary psychology – which attempts to work out human and animal behaviour in evolutionary terms. In the foreword to one of the classic books on this subject, *The Selfish Gene* by evolutionary biologist Richard Dawkins, Trivers explains why animals might have evolved the power of self-deceit. According to Trivers, animals would have evolved the ability to recognize when another animal was being deceitful; then, like an evolutionary arms race, the deceitful animals may have evolved mechanisms that lead to self-deception. This would 'render some facts and motives unconscious, so as not to betray – by subtle signs of self-knowledge – the deception being practised'.

Trivers believes that the different roles of the two cerebral hemispheres are apparent when a person is being deceitful – that we are still able to detect deceit, despite the proposed evolution of self-deceit that is supposed to mask it. 'If you put a false expression on your face – a forced smile – it will tend to curl up a bit more on the right side of the face, because it is being run by the left hemisphere. The right hemisphere is more involved in a natural expression, so if I could smile warmly at you now, it is supposed to curl up a bit more on the left side, because it is run by the right brain.' He has analysed video footage of President Bill Clinton discussing his alleged sexual relations with a woman who was working at the White House. In the face of this scandal, Clinton lied to the media: 'I did not have sexual relations with that woman.' Trivers says that when Clinton was denying his involvement with the woman, he subconsciously showed the signs of deceit in the imbalance between the two sides of his face. 'Initially, there was a facial imbalance – the right face was into it, the left face said, "Get me the hell out of here".' Trivers notes that the balance was redressed when Clinton eventually went before the media to admit that he had lied; both sides of his face were 'into it'. Ramachandran agrees: 'Your face starts leaking traces of deceit ... the muscles are slightly different when you are lying.'

We have seen that the strange lack of awareness of the left-hand side of the world evident in visual-neglect patients, and the denial of symptoms in anosagnosic patients, are caused by damage to the right parietal lobe. Earlier, we saw that the equally curious symptoms of blind-sight patients is caused by damage to the visual cortex in the occipital lobes. Broca's aphasia is one example of the results of damage sustained in the frontal lobe. That leaves the temporal lobes – what might damage to them be able to tell us about their function?

The temporal lobes are tucked in almost underneath the rest of the brain, right behind the ears and the temples. As you might expect, their proximity to the ears means that the temporal lobes are heavily involved in our sense of hearing. Just as there are sensory maps of the body on the parietal lobes, motor maps of the body on the frontal lobes and retinal maps on the occipital lobes, there are auditory maps on the temporal lobes. The cortex here is arranged according to the frequency of a sound, so that two closely pitched notes will stimulate adjacent areas. The temporal lobes are also involved in efforts to understand or recognize sounds. Adjacent to the auditory maps is an area of association cortex. Sometimes, damage to the auditory association cortex results in auditory agnosia. A person affected by this strange dysfunction can hear sounds, but does not recognize them. Also in the temporal lobes, just behind the auditory association areas, lie regions of association cortex involved in visual recognition. And just as auditory agnosia is the result of damage to auditory association cortex, damage to the visual association cortex can cause visual agnosia – the inability to recognize objects by sight.

What are you looking at?

In the 1970s Philip was injured in a serious road traffic accident which put him into a coma for several weeks. Luckily, he regained consciousness and his brain seemed to be functioning normally, despite the force of the collision. It was soon realized that Philip had sustained damage to part of his temporal lobe near to the back of the brain: the visual association cortex. The result of this damage is that Philip has trouble recognizing animals and fruit and vegetables. His neurologist, Dr Rosalind McCarthy, shows him a photograph of King's College Chapel in Cambridge, and asks him if he can identify it. Philip replies, 'That's King's College' – he can recognize buildings. He can find his way around, too, and he picks his daughter up from school every day. When shown a pair of scissors, a pair of glasses and a toy helicopter, Philip names them immediately. However, when McCarthy shows Philip a toy elephant, Philip has no idea what it is. He says, 'It's an endangered species but I can't place it, though. I tell you what gives it away to me are the tusks at the front, and I know what it is but I can't name it. It's annoying me.'

At the zoo, standing next to the giraffe enclosure, he says that the giraffes might just as well be extinct dinosaurs or the Loch Ness monster. In the end, he guesses that the animals he can see must be camels – because he had heard passers-by talking about camels, which are in the enclosure behind him. He eventually discovers that the animals he is looking at are giraffes by reading a sign alongside the enclosure. Philip always looks out for clues like these when identifying objects that he does not immediately recognize. And when a pineapple is held in front of his face, he is equally unable to name it. When the pineapple is handed to him, he correctly states that 'it grows on trees, comes from hot climates, it's juicy, you can't eat the outside' – then 'I've forgotten what it is.' It seems sensible that normal human vision has the ability to draw associations between objects that it sees. This sort of information, which seems to emerge subconsciously and from different, undamaged parts of the brain, is important for survival. Some patients with more extensive temporal lobe damage have trouble even with this kind of subconscious recognition: they put just about anything into their mouths, even razor blades or the wrong end of a lit cigarette. This kind of associated knowledge would have been even more important to pre-historic hunter–gatherers – as would the ability to recall associated knowledge about animals, which could have been predator or prey, for example, or fruit that could be poisonous or nutritious. Philip can function at this subcon-scious level, but has trouble simply extending his recognition of objects by name.

Philip's agnosia includes the inability to recognize faces, a condition known as prosopagnosia. This is the same condition that 'LH' suffered from, as described in 'Mind Readers'. When shown a photograph of Margaret Thatcher, Philip cannot name her. When shown a photo-graph of the late Princess Diana, he guesses who it is by looking at her earrings. Marilyn Monroe and Elvis Presley are the subjects of the next photographs, and Philip has no idea who they are. When asked whether he knows who Elvis Presley is, he explains that Presley was a famous American singer and film actor who made his mark in the 1950s, and who is now dead. When he tries to conjure up an image of

Elvis, he sees sequins, but does not know why. When meeting familiar people, he can only recognize them by the sound of their voice or their 'habits, clothes, hairstyles, nose, moustache'. When Ramachandran draws a picture of Donald Duck on a white board, Philip has no idea who it is. He guesses that it might be the late Grace Kelly.

People have long suspected that parts of the temporal lobes are heavily involved in the recognition of faces, but only recently have neurophysiologists begun working out the extent of the role of the temporal lobes in the recognition of other objects. Blakemore and his colleague Tim Andrews at Oxford University are among a number of researchers carrying out imaging studies, using fMRI, aiming to discover which parts of the cortex are involved in visual recognition. Some other researchers are using a more direct method of spying on the brain: by connecting electrodes to the cortex of a living monkey, they can find out at precisely which point the cortex is active when the monkey is engaged in various specific visual tasks.

Philip's 'category-specific' agnosia has affected only very limited aspects of his vision: his ability to recognize animals, fruit and vegetables and faces. This suggests that vision actually consists of a number of different modules, each with a particular job. Until the 1960s it was thought that the visual pathways from the retina led only to the maps on the visual cortex in the occipital lobes. The problem with this idea is that it does not explain our experience of seeing. In fact, the classic idea that the optic nerve leads to the cortex and perceived there is not too far away from an idea by the French philosopher René Descartes in the sixteenth century.

Descartes cut away the retina of a disembodied sheep's eye and replaced it with a translucent screen. He found that the lens in the eye produced an image of his window on the screen, and he correctly surmised that the retina is a simple screen, too. Descartes supposed that the optic nerve carried the image from the retina deep into the brain, where it produced another image. The soul could then view the scene. Many people today think in a similar way – unable to conceive of a way that the tissues of the brain could be responsible for the awareness of actually seeing something. Instead, many believe that there is a soul or spirit that does the seeing – just as Descartes did. However, this does not explain how vision works, because it does not explain how the soul sees. For some people, the soul takes on human form, so that there is a little person inside your head who does the seeing. Professor Ramachandran says that if the image is simply projected inside the brain for a little person to see it, then that little person must have another brain, with another person inside it. He says, 'You end up with an infinite regress of eyes and images and little people without solving the problem of perception.'

The rich experience of vision is many-faceted. Among its many functions are spatial awareness and avoidance of obstacles, reaching and grabbing things, general awareness, communication and the recognition of objects (Philip's problem). The brain needs to interpret colour, form, shape, a sense of space; it needs to search its database of associated memories about an object; it must be able to follow smooth movement of an object across its visual field. As you would expect with so many different functions, there are many different areas of the brain involved in vision.

We have seen that the visual information from the retinas enters the brain along two main pathways: an older one and a newer one. The older pathway – involved in visual reflexes and a sense of space – terminates in the parietal lobes, as discussed above. The new pathway leads through the thalamus to the visual cortex, and is involved in conscious awareness. In a sense, the visual cortex in the occipital lobes is like the hypothetical screen described above – it is a simple map of the visual field. Other areas of the brain interpret what is 'displayed' there, and each area carries out a different, well-defined operation on the information it receives. More than thirty such areas have so far been identified, with specializations for sensing colour, movement, relative distance and depth, the form, movement and orientation of objects. Despite this thirty-fold division of labour, the visual functions of the brain seem to follow two distinct pathways from the visual cortex. The first of these is referred to as the 'where pathway' or the 'how pathway', and is concerned with enabling you to work out the location and distance of objects, and with finding your way around and avoiding obstacles. The 'how' pathway shares some of the functions of the evolutionarily ancient pathway that blindsight patients rely on to invoke unconscious responses to visual information. And, like that ancient visual pathway, it ends up in the parietal lobe. In Philip, the 'how' pathway is clearly undamaged, since he can walk – and even drive – around in the world as well as anyone. However, the 'what' pathway for visual information – involved in visual recognition – is what is damaged in him.

When Philip is handling a piece of fruit, he can call up associations with that fruit, as he did with the pineapple. In this case, his subconscious brain systems know what type of fruit he is handling, but this information cannot be interpreted using his higher-level functions, like language and memory. Colin Blakemore explains that part of the 'what' pathway is involved in condensing the information about the world 'into a succinct description which becomes a memory ... and second, to use that same kind of description as the basis of language ... a word is a wonderful symbol'. Surprising evidence of the role of the temporal lobes in memory is that stimulation of the auditory association cortex in awake patients undergoing brain surgery evokes complex memories of sounds. Visual memories can be evoked by stimulation of the same area, in certain patients. The 'what' pathway – involving the temporal lobes – is involved in recognition of objects, and it is this pathway that is damaged in Philip. More tantalizing evidence about the function of the 'what' pathway comes from another curious syndrome, called Capgras' syndrome.

A case of mistaken identity

After a road accident a few years ago a young man, David, suffered damage to his temporal lobes. He was in a coma for a week but, when he regained consciousness, his behaviour showed no real ill effects. He was not psychotic or emotionally disturbed, but he was suffering from one remarkable delusion: that his mother and father were impostors. He agreed that they looked identical to his real parents, but he simply would not accept that they were who they said they were. David's mother recalls the events of one meal time: 'He probably didn't like the food that day, because he said, "That lady who comes in the morning, she cooks much better than you" ... but the lady was me all the time.' Speaking about his father, David explains, 'He can look like my father but the fact is that it doesn't feel like him because I know that it is not him.' David's disbelief about the identity of his parents is so strong that he does not re-cognize the family home. One day, he demanded to be taken to his real home. His mother took him out of the apartment building, around the block, and returned to the same apartment, where she left him alone. In the absence of the supposed impostors, David was then satisfied that this really was home. David's symptoms are known by the name Capgras' syndrome or Capgras' delusion.

Capgras' syndrome was first reported during the early years of the twentieth century. Until recently, the textbook explanation of its strange symptoms has been based on one of Sigmund Freud's ideas – the Oedipus complex. The explan-ation goes something like this: Freud claimed that sexual feelings are felt by a son towards his mother, or a daughter towards her father, in early childhood. These feelings are repressed as a child develops and, in a normal adult, there is no sexual attraction to parents. In certain people, those repressed feelings come to the surface in adulthood, causing unrest in a person's personality. This is the Oedipus complex. According to the Freudian interpretation of Capgras' syndrome, the damage sustained by the patients' brains somehow releases the sexual feelings towards their parent – the Oedipus complex brought on by a nasty knock on the head. The patient is then aware of sexual feelings towards someone who looks just like his or her parent. The brain subconsciously deals with this: it convinces its belief system to assume that this person is not a parent after all.

There are certain reasons why this interpretation does not work, including the fact that the Oedipus complex involves sexual feelings only towards the parent of the opposite sex. David denies the identity of his father as well as his mother. Furthermore, it is not only parents that are the subject of the delusions experienced in Capgras' syndrome. Often it will be a wife or a husband. Ramachandran has even seen a patient who has the same delusion about his dog: 'He'll look at his pet dog and say, "Doctor, this is not Fifi. It looks like Fifi, but it's been replaced by an identical dog."' The Oedipus complex cannot really explain that particular case.

Ramachandran has suggested an alternative explanation of Capgras' syndrome, which appeals to recent advances in understanding the 'what' pathway of the visual system. There are connections between the areas of the temporal lobes involved in recognition – the ones that were damaged in Philip – and the limbic system, which is the emotional centre of the brain. In particular, there are major connections to the amygdalae, whose roles were discussed in 'Mind Readers'. The amygdalae are heavily involved in producing emotional responses, in creating feelings about things. Ramachandran explains: 'When you look at an object, the message goes first to your temporal lobe cortex, where you recognize it ... after you've recognized it, you also need to respond to it emotionally.' This is probably important in our appreciation of great works of art, but it must have developed – back in our evolutionary history – as a mechanism to avoid danger or to find a mate. Seeing a looming predator makes an animal feel differently from how it feels when it sees a mate, and the animal responds accordingly. This seems to be true of humans, too: laboratory tests show that a person's body sweats very slightly when that person sees something that evokes an emotional response. The emotions can be almost imperceptible, but the sweating response can be recorded, as a change in the GSR (galvanic skin response), after a few seconds. The GSR is a measurement of the skin's conductivity – how well it conducts electricity – and is determined by attaching electrodes to a person's palm, where the sweating is most pronounced.

Ramachandran proposes that a specific part of David's 'what' pathway was damaged in his accident – the part that connects the temporal lobe with the amygdalae. When David looks at his mother, his temporal lobe recognizes her and brings forth appropriate memories. But David's temporal lobes do not communicate with his amygdalae, because the connection is broken. So there is recognition of faces, but not the expected feelings that should accompany that recognition. To make sense of the conflict between the visual memory and the lack of emotion, David's brain – perhaps his storytelling left parietal lobe – works out that this person must be an impostor. There is evidence to support this idea. First, strong connections between the temporal lobes and the limbic system do exist – clearly there is communication between the recognition centres of the temporal lobes and the emotional centres of the limbic system. Also, David has no problem accepting his parents' identity when he can only hear them – over the telephone, for example. The Freudian explanation does not seem to fit in with that observation. The connection between the auditory cortex – also in the temporal lobe – and the amygdalae is separate from the one that connects the visual association cortex to the amygdalae.

To test his idea, Ramachandran and his colleagues decided to measure David's GSR while he was shown a series of photographs of people's faces. Some of the photographs showed total strangers, while the others showed his mother and father. Normal people produce a GSR when they look at photographs of their parents – 'Every time you look at your mother, you start sweating,' says Ramachandran. If his theory is correct about the disconnection between the temporal lobe and the amygdalae, then you would expect no response when David sees photographs of his parents. And that is exactly what he found. It seems to show how closely our intellect is linked to basic emotional reactions.

Ramachandran accepts that his theory cannot explain all aspects of Capgras' syndrome. It does not explain why the syndrome is normally restricted to a patient's parents or spouse, for example. Another Capgras' syndrome patient is Oliver, who is delusional only about his wife. 'I thought it was a twin of her,' he says. In fact, Oliver was convinced that his wife was three different people. His delusions led him to believe that one of the people who claimed to be his wife was spying on him to gather information for the other two. Oliver's neurologist is Dr Simon Fleminger of Goldsmiths College, London University. Like Ramachandran, Fleminger believes that the physiological explanation of Capgras' syndrome is not enough. He suggests that a psychological dimension is necessary to explain the syndrome. He says, 'There is a to-and-fro between the information coming from the outside world on the one hand, and our thoughts of what we are about to see on the other ... Our expectations can colour what we perceive.' Oliver's delusion may be caused by his belief that his wife is not to be trusted, which then affects his perception of his wife.

So it seems that the emotional responses of the limbic system feed into the areas of the temporal lobes involved in recognition – how you feel about something can help you to identify it. A dramatic illustration of the relationship between emotions and the temporal lobes is found in epileptic seizures that occur in the temporal lobes.

A religious experience

In Capgras' syndrome, it seems that the connections between the temporal lobes and the amygdalae are disrupted, so that the patient does not feel the appropriate emotional response when looking at a familiar face. Ramachandran believes that a well-known effect in patients who have epileptic seizures in their temporal lobes is the opposite: such people can see emotional significance in almost everything, and often declare themselves to be modern-day prophets or visionaries.

An epileptic seizure is like an avalanche of electrical signals in the brain. Ramachandran describes an epileptic seizure as like an 'electrical storm in the brain; where a group of neurones starts discharging, unco-ordinated from the rest of the brain'. The increase in electrical activity can produce extreme convulsions, during which the whole body begins to shake violently, and a person loses consciousness. Less severe or more localized seizures can cause just one part of the body to shake or can result in a momentary loss of awareness.

The close connection between the temporal lobe and the limbic system – of which the amygdalae are part – explains why seizures localized in the temporal lobes are likely to evoke strong emotional responses. The limbic system is also responsible for emotional response to the sense of smell, and to memory and hearing. During a seizure in the temporal lobe, patients often have visions and hear voices, and sometimes sense noxious smells or tastes. A sense of déjà vu is also fairly common in temporal-lobe seizures. One experience that has been reported by some patients with temporal-lobe epilepsy, since it was first studied a hundred years or so ago, is a religious feeling. This can manifest itself as a visitation by God, or the belief that the patients actually are God. Amid the disrupting of bodily functions – often including a disturbing physical fit – there is a sense of understanding the world, a spiritual high, like being at one with the cosmos.

One patient who suffers from temporal-lobe epilepsy is John, who separates the physical dimension of the seizures from the 'spiritual' dimension. 'The seizures involve my person – that's the seizure I'm experiencing – and my soul, and my spirit,' he says. John actually welcomes the spiritual feelings that he experiences: 'You're fighting with your soul and your spirit afterwards.' Describing a recent seizure, he explains that, 'My attitude was that I was God, and I had heaven and hell in my eyes. You know, I was the grand guy who created heaven and hell.' Sometimes, John has seven or eight seizures in a single day, each one lasting between three and six minutes. During each one, he is in another realm: 'through the gateway and into another reality'. The experiences of temporal-lobe epilepsy are extremely real, and they can be extremely emotional. In tears, John gives an idea of the intensity of his experiences: 'I've been in so much pain that I would rather be shot or whipped to death; and yet I've been in so much joy that I would rather be left alone; take everything away and just let me sit there, and have that much joy … I feel like I can float, it's the best.' Before John had his first seizure, at the age of seventeen, he was a normal adolescent, and was not religious. In Ancient Greece epilepsy was known as 'the sacred disease'. In some cultures in Asia, India and Australia, people who suffer from epilepsy are thought to be in contact with a transcendent reality, and therefore able to heal or foretell the future. They may become shamans – the word 'shaman' means 'he who knows'. John believes he has special insight: 'I am so right in my own head, I know I could go out there and get people to follow me … Were all the prophets people who were flopping around on the ground? Is that was this whole message was, this whole time?'

In his book *Phantoms in the Brain* Ramachandran describes a device called a transcranial magnetic stimulator, which is a helmet that can be used to excite any part of the brain. He describes a Canadian neuroscientist, Professor Michael Persinger, who used one of these devices to stimulate his temporal lobes. He was attempting to instil within himself the sort of experience that John has during his temporal lobe seizures, and he succeeded. In his 1987 book *The Neuropsychological Base of God Beliefs* he investigated the origins of religious beliefs. He has also suggested how UFO sightings may be explained by hallucination. In each case, he looked for the source of the psychological experience in terms of the physiological brain. Ramachandran, too, has devised a physiological explanation of why even atheists can have seemingly religious experiences during a temporal-lobe seizure.

According to Ramachandran, the importance of the amygdalae in the creation of emotions and their proximity to the temporal lobes means that seizures in the temporal lobes will produce a welling up of a huge range of emotions. The brain's normal emotional response to the world is important, and is to some extent 'hard-wired': the reactions to aggression, for example, are important for survival. The emotional responses of the limbic system are not all hardwired, however. We develop our own personal emotional reactions, to things that have certain meanings to us. Ramachandran says that we create a 'landscape of emotional salience' in the barrage of different emotions experienced during temporal-lobe epileptic seizures. And repeated seizures can produce permanent changes to the emotional pathways – a process called kindling. Ramachandran proposes that kindling along the pathways between the temporal lobes and the amygdalae is what brings the sensations of glory, so that almost anything can be imbued with emotional significance.

This tendency to assign significance to everyday objects might relate to mystical experience. John's father reports, 'When he has had a seizure he'll want to talk philosophy. He'll want to discuss all the things that are floating around in the stew he's got up here that he's trying to reconstruct.' Religious beliefs are widespread, occurring in every human society, and they can contribute to social stability. Collective worship or shared belief in a supreme being can bring a group of people together, for example. Ramachandran stresses that if the source of religious or spiritual feelings is physiological, this does not undermine or devalue such feelings. He says that they can enrich the patient's life. This poses a dilemma for neurologists: 'What right do we have to treat the patient with medication or with surgery, thereby depriving him of these valuable experiences that often enrich his mental life?' The experiences of patients with temporal-lobe epilepsy may be related to creativity, too. There is evidence that the Dutch artist Vincent van Gogh suffered from temporal-lobe epilepsy, in which case he would have experienced heightened emotional responses to visual images. This may go some way to explaining his emotionally charged, visionary paintings and his delusional mental state.

Opening up the brain

In years gone by, people who claimed that their parents were impostors, believed they were prophets or denied the existence of their medical conditions were usually simply labelled 'mad'. One of the positive things to come from the study of the brain is the potential for understanding strange behaviours like these in terms of physiology. In particular, as we have seen, study of the effects of damage to the most complex part of the brain – the cerebrum – may explain some of the most bizarre things that can happen to the human mind. Ramachandran is excited about the fact that subjects such as creativity, God and religion – once the exclusive province of psychology, theology, philosophy and metaphysics – can now be studied in terms of the physiology of the brain. Consciousness, too – while still elusive to neuroscientists – may one day be understood in terms of signals dashing around the brain, just as memories, emotion and perception are being understood today. As more and more of the incredible behaviours and abilities of the human mind come under study in terms of the brain's hardware, we may be moving closer to the day when the human brain can understand itself.

AFTERWORD
. . .looking ahead. . .

Neuroscience is moving forwards ever more rapidly. From a philosophical point of view, it is working towards the same goal as the Human Genome Project, cosmology and the study of evolution: the understanding of the very nature of ourselves. On a more practical level, neuroscience holds out hope for people suffering from conditions such as epilepsy, Parkinson's disease and schizophrenia. Most strategies to overcome or correct diseases or disorders of the nervous system are currently based around drugs or the removal of or deliberate damage to parts of the brain during surgery. The surgical approach to treating diseases or disorders of the brain is often carried out while the patient is awake, since only then can surgeons be sure they are in the desired spot in which they can destroy or remove an area of brain tissue. Although this sort of operation has been carried out for decades, and is growing in success rate and sophistication, it is still an arduous and delicate procedure for patient and surgeon, and does not always work. In the future, when scientific understanding of the brain is far more accomplished, surgery may be more accurate, consistent and free from side effects.

In the long-term future, however, the best treatment of brain damage or deficiency may be the combination of the 'wet' brain and 'dry' silicon-based electronics. Scientists have already managed to connect brain cells to semi-conductors such as silicon, and the development of a 'brain expansion chip' may not be too far into the future. It could perhaps replace areas of brain tissue lost to disease or in accidents. This kind of approach may also one day give sight to some blind people: connecting a light-sensitive electronic chip like that found in a video camera to a patient's optic nerve has already been attempted, with some encouraging results. This is just one of a number of different approaches to helping blind people see again. Neuroscience is changing our relationship with our brains. In the future, paralysis, blindness, deafness, loss of memory, learning disabilities – all of these may be overcome using what will become routine treatment.

Perhaps just as important as the potential neurological treatments is the fact that discovering the pathology – the nature and causes – of brain disorders allows us to understand people with unusual behaviour or strange mental disabilities. Autism, once thought to be the product of bad parenting, is now understood in terms of what goes on in the autistic brain: it is no longer blamed on parents or on the children themselves. People who suffer from schizophrenia or epilepsy are better understood, too. With understanding can come compassion and tolerance.

Understanding how the brain works, how it develops and how it determines behaviour could also have its downside: it might enable people wielding political or economic power to control or manipulate minds, or to discriminate against others. Advertising companies and media-hungry politicians – already often powerful forces in behaviour modification by tapping into our subconscious fears and desires – could launch even more successful offensives on the minds of humans as consumers and voters, armed with sophisticated knowledge about the brain.

The revolution in genetics is also a potential threat to liberty. The modern techniques used by geneticists might enable them to locate particular versions of genes that occur more often in people with certain types of personality than in others. Genes that influence the following behaviours and abilities have all been located: intelligence, depression, alcoholism, thrill seeking and homosexuality (though this is in dispute), as well as a number of congenital brain disorders. In the very near future, scientists will have completed the Human Genome Project – the detailed map of all the genes possessed by human beings. The links between genes and behaviour will be much easier to track down, but perhaps also to change or select. Indeed, one day it may be possible to choose certain behavioural aspects as well as physical characteristics in an unborn child by manipulating the human genome. For example, parents may want an incredibly intelligent baby, or one that is good at languages or musically gifted. For now, this is just over the border from reality, into science fiction. But it may not be too far into the future before it becomes part of reality. Many people are deeply concerned about this possibility, and the spectre of 'designer babies'.

What might the future hold for the study of the brain and behaviour? Perhaps the twenty-first century will bring artificial brain implants, intelligent robots, more consistent and wide-ranging brain surgery, new ways of learning and hyper-intelligent children. However, it may be longer than we think before neuroscience can bring any of these technological marvels, and a radically new view of ourselves: many commentators suggest that neuroscience is at a similar stage of development today as physics and chemistry were around the middle of the nineteenth century. If this is true, then we must recognize how limited our understanding may be, and how some of the currently accepted theories about the brain may be seen as primitive in a hundred years or so. And even then, there will still be many mysteries – just as there still are today with both physics and chemistry.

In fact it is unlikely that we shall ever be able to solve all the mysteries of the brain. The more we discover about the brain, the more we realize there is still to discover. Emerson Pugh, a pioneer researcher into artificial intelligence computer systems, once remarked, 'If the human brain were simple enough to understand, we'd be so simple we wouldn't be able to understand it.'

GLOSSARY

amygdalae   Structures in the brain involved in generating emotional responses, such as fear. They are sometimes considered to be part of the limbic system. There are two amygdalae.

auditory cortex   The part of the cerebrum at which signals from the ear arrive.

axon   A long fibre that is part of a neurone, and along which nerve signals pass within the brain and the nervous system in general.

brainstem   The part of the brain that connects to the spinal cord. Signals to and from the body pass through it – and cross over in it, which is why each cerebral hemisphere is associated with the opposite side of the body.

cerebellum   The 'little brain' at the back of the brain, near the top of the brainstem. It is involved in co-ordination and in keeping the muscles toned.

cerebral hemisphere   One of the two large sections of the cerebrum. The left cerebral hemisphere is more concerned with language and mathematics, the right with spatial awareness and creative ability.

cerebrospinal fluid (CSF)
The liquid, produced in the ventricles, which surrounds the brain and spinal cord. The brain is effectively floating in CSF, and this reduces its weight. CSF also cushions the brain during an impact, protecting it from injury.

cerebrum
The largest part of the brain, associated with its higher processes. The cerebrum consists of two cerebral hemispheres, each divided into four lobes. The outer layer of the cerebrum is the cortex.

chromosome
One of the DNA-containing objects in the nucleus of a cell. Humans have forty-six chromosomes in all, including two chromosomes that determine an individual's sex.

corpus callosum
The large, dense bundle of nerve fibres that connects the two cerebral hemispheres.

cortex
The grey outer layer of the cerebrum. There are three different types of cortex: sensory, motor and association.

dendrite
One of the many slender fibres that emanate from a neurone. Dendrites form synapses with other neurones, so that signals from the other neurones can pass to the dendrite and into the neurone of which it is part.

deoxyribonucleic acid (DNA)	Deoxyribonucleic acid, a chemical substance found in chromosomes, which carries information from generation to generation. That information relates to body characteristics, but may also affect behaviour.
hippocampus	Part of the limbic system that is involved in generating emotional responses. There are two hippocampi.
hormone	A chemical messenger that helps to regulate various bodily functions. Many hormones are produced in the brain, by the hypothalamus and the pituitary gland.
hypothalamus	A structure in the brain, literally 'below the thalamus', which produces hormones that regulate body temperature, hunger and thirst, sexual behaviour and aggression. It is closely associated with the limbic system, and most of the hormones the hypothalamus produces directly affect the pituitary gland.
intelligence quotient (IQ)	A number derived from psychometric tests that purport to measure general intelligence. It is standardized, so that the average IQ of a large number of people is 100.

limbic system   A collection of structures in the brain that lie to either side of the centre, and are involved in generating emotional responses and also in producing memories. Its structures include the hippocampus and the amygdalae.

meninges   Three membranes that enclose the brain and the spinal cord. Inflammation of the meninges is called meningitis.

magnetic resonance imaging (MRI)   A technique used to produce images of a living brain without having to open the skull. Functional MRI (fMRI) can show which parts of the brain are working the hardest during a particular task.

neurone   The fundamental unit of the nervous system. It is composed of a cell body, from which axons and dendrites originate.

neurotransmitter   A chemical substance in the brain whose release from an axon facilitates the transmission of a nerve signal across a synapse.

orbito-frontal cortex   Part of the frontal lobe of the cerebrum associated with personality, in particular social behaviour.

pituitary gland   A small organ, located just behind the nasal passage, which produces a range of important hormones. Most of its functions are controlled by the hypothalamus.

positron emission tomography (PET)   A technique used to produce images of a living brain without opening the skull.

psychometrics   Tests that aim to measure aspects of behaviour, such as IQ.

receptor   A cell or group of cells that responds to a stimulus, such as light, pressure or a change in temperature. The dendrites of a sensory neurone form synapses with receptors, and carry a signal from a stimulated receptor to the spinal cord or to the brain.

synapse   A tiny gap between the dendrite of one neurone and the axon of another. Neurotransmitters released at one side stimulate a nerve signal to jump across the synaptic gap.

thalamus   Part of the brain that relays sensory information from the head and body to the relevant part of the cortex. There are two thalami.

ventricle   A space inside the brain in which cerebrospinal fluid is produced.

visual cortex   Part of the cortex on the occipital lobe of each cerebral hemisphere. Signals produced by receptors in the retinas of the eyes arrive at the visual cortex after passing through the thalamus.

SELECTED BIBLIOGRAPHY

Mind Readers

Baron-Cohen, Simon, and Patrick Bolton, *Autism*, Oxford Paperbacks, Oxford, 1993.

Frith, Uta, *Autism*, Blackwell Publishers, Oxford, 1989.

Rosner, Eleanor, and Sue R. Semel, *Williams' Syndrome*, Blackwell Publishers, Oxford, 1998.

Sacks, Oliver, *An Anthropologist on Mars*, Picador, London, 1995.

Scariano, Margaret M., *Emergence: Labelled Autistic – Temple Gradin*, Warner Books, New York, 1996.

Natural-born Genius

Devlin, Bernie (ed.) and Stephen E. Fienberg, *Intelligence, Genes, and Success: Scientists Respond to The Bell Curve*, Copernicus Books, New York, 1997.

Eysenck, Hans J., *Intelligence: The New Look*, Transaction Publishers, New Brunswick, 1998.

Gardner, Howard, Mindy Kornhaber and Warren Wake, *Intelligence: Multiple Perspectives*, Harcourt Publishers Ltd, New York, 1996.

Herrnstein, Richard J., and Charles Murray, *The Bell Curve: Intelligence and Class Structure in American Life*, The Free Press (a division of Simon and Schuster), New York, 1994.

Kinchloe, Joe L. and Shirley R. Steinberg (eds), and Aaron d'Gresson, *Measured Lies: The Bell Curve Examined*, St Martin's Press, New York, 1996.

Phantom Brains

Melzack, Ronald, and Patrick D. Wall, *The Challenge of Pain*, Penguin Books, London, 1993.

Ramachandran, V. S., and Sandra Blakeslee, *Phantoms in the Brain*, Fourth Estate Ltd, London, 1998 (paperback 1999).

Living Dangerously

Bernstein, Peter L., *Against the Gods: The Remarkable Story of Risk*, John Wiley and Sons, New York, 1996.

Tomlinson, Joe, *The Ultimate Encyclopedia of Extreme Sports*, Carlton Books, London, 1996.

Wilde, Gerald J. S., *Target Risk*, PDE Publications, Toronto, 1995.

Willis, Jim, Albert A. Okunade and William J. Willis, *Reporting on Risks*, Praeger Pub Text, Westport, Connecticut, 1997.

Zuckerman, Marvin (ed.), *Behavioral Expression and Biosocial Bases of Sensation Seeking*, Cambridge University Press, Cambridge, 1994.

Thin Air

Boukreev, Anatoli, and G. Watson Dewalt, *The Climb: Tragic Ambitions on Everest*, St Martin's Press, New York, 1998.

Krakauer, Jon, *Into Thin Air*, Random House, New York, 1998.

Lieberman, Philip, *Eve Spoke: Human Language and Human Evolution*, Macmillan Publishers Ltd, London, 1998.

Phillips, John L., *The Bends: Compressed Air in the History of Science, Diving and Engineering*, Yale University Press, Newhaven, Connecticut, 1998.

Lies and Delusions

Freeman, Walter J., *How Brains Make Up Their Minds*, Weidenfeld & Nicolson General, London, 1999.

Sacks, Oliver, *The Man Who Mistook His Wife for a Hat*, HarperCollins, New York, 1986.

Weiskrantz, Lawrence, *Consciousness Lost and Found*, Oxford University Press, Oxford, 1998.

General

Cairns-Smith, A. G., *Secrets of the Mind: A Tale of Discovery and Mistaken Identity*, Springer Verlag New York Inc, New York, 1999.

Carter, Rita, and Christopher Frith, *Mapping the Mind*, Weidenfeld Illustrated, London, 1998.

Greenfield, Susan, *The Human Brain: A Guided Tour*, Weidenfield & Nicolson, London, 1997 (paperback 1998: Phoenix, a division of Orion Books).

Ridley, Matt, *Genome: The Autobiography of a Species in 23 Chapters*, Fourth Estate, London, 1999.

INDEX

Howe, Michael 66
Hubel, David 102–3
Human Genome Project 50, 54, 79, 221
Humboldt, Alexander von 159–60
humours 130
Huxley, Aldous 82
hyperbaric chambers 161, 162–3, 172
hyperventilation 163–4
hypothalamus 11, 25, 26, 108
hypoxia 157, 158–9, 165, 170, 172, 176, 180
    see also altitude sickness
hypoxic ventilatory response (HVR) 164

I
imipramine 140
imprinting 44–5
insulin-like growth factor 2 receptor (IGF2R) 80–1
intelligence 14, 49–83
    Asperger's syndrome 27–8
    autism 29, 34
    definition 54
    quotient (IQ) 56, 58, 60, 62, 67–9, 71–6
    social 47–8
    testing 54–66, 73–6
Iowa State University 77
iproniazid 140
Irvine, Sandy 168
isocarboxazid 140

J
Jangbu Sherpar 150, 178
Jessel, David 21
Johanson, Richard 123
Jung, Carl 130, 131, 132

K
Kanner, Leo 27
Kates, Wendy 37
Kemper, Thomas 37
King, David 52, 61

L
Lacoste-Utamsing, Christine De 23
lateral geniculate nucleus 189
Lavoisier, Antoine-Laurent 153–4
leaky gut 28
LeDoux, Joseph 37
Libet, Benjamin 200
Lieberman, Philip 158
limbic system 11, 36, 97, 144, 211, 212, 214, 216
lobotomy 39–40
lungs 154–5, 157, 159, 161, 171

M
McCarthy, Rosalind 205
McGuffin, Peter 78
mad cow disease 124
magnetic resonance imaging (MRI) 14, 36, 37, 38, 156, 163–4, 179, 180
    see also functional magnetic resonance imaging (fMRI)
magnetoencephalography (MEG) 105–6, 112
Mallory, George 168
Malpighi, Marcello 12
Mauna Kea 152
medulla 170
Melzack, Ronald 96–8, 109–10, 114, 115
Mendel, Gregor 70–1
Merzenich, Michael 100–1
Messner, Reinhold 174
Milner, Peter 144
mind reading 17–48
Minnesota Study 69
mirror box 109–10, 113
mirrors 190, 193
Mitchell, Silus Weir 87
Moir, Anne 21
molecular genetics 50
Monge's disease 171
monoamine oxidase (MAO) 139–42, 145, 146
monoamine oxidase type B (MAO B) 133–7, 141
motor cortex 184, 196
motor neurones 89

pre-eclampsia 123
Priestley, Joseph 153
projective tests 131
prosopagnosia 206
Prozac 140
psychology 10, 130–3
psychometric testing 65–6,
    165–6, 172–3, 175, 176, 177,
    178–9, 180
    see also intelligence testing
Pugh, Emerson 222
pulmonary oedema 171, 172,
    175
pulse oxymeter 169, 172, 176,
    179
Pythagoras 11

R
race, intelligence 74–5
Rain Man 29
Ramachandran, Vilayanur
    192–4, 198, 199–200, 201,
    202–3, 204, 207, 208
    Capgras' syndrome 211–13
    epilepsy 214, 216
    phantom limbs 103–7,
        108–10, 113–14
    religion 217, 218
    visual neglect 192–4
reaction times 55–6, 66
readiness potential 200
referred pain 91
relativity 201
respiration 154, 155–6, 161
restriction fragment length
    polymorphism 79
retina 189, 207–8
reward cascade 144
reward deficiency syndrome
    146
reward pathways 143–4, 145
rhizotomy 94, 100
risk 117–47
    Risk Homeostasis Theory
        119, 120
Rosenbaum, Gail 165, 166,
    180

S
saccades 190–1
Sacks, Oliver 30–1
Sally-Anne Test 33–4, 35
Scarr, Sandra 67, 82
Scheele, Karl 153
schizophrenia 28, 138, 220
Schoene, Brownie 163–4
seat belts 119, 120–1
Seese, Nicole 78
self 183–4, 198–205
self-awareness 190
Sensation Seeking Scale 133,
    141
sensory cortex 184, 196
sensory neurones 89
serotonin 28, 29, 115, 138, 139,
    140
sex chromosomes 42, 43–6
sex dimorphism 23–6
sexual orientation 25
sexual stereotypes 20–3
shared attention 32
Sherpa people 168
skin colour 72
Skinner, Burrhus F. 130, 131
Skuse, David 41, 42, 43–5, 47
social brain 17–48
soul 208
Spearman, Charles 59, 61, 64
spectrum disorders 27
speech 158, 185
Sperry, Roger 196
spinal cord 89
spirometry 164
split-brain patients 196–7
Staker, Jay 77
stereotypes, sexual 20–3
Stern, William 58
strokes 160, 187, 192
Stroop test 165–6
superior colliculus 190, 191, 199
synaptic gaps 138

T
Tager-Flusberg, Helen 34–5
Taub, Edward 100

5